Cynthia Daddona

Hypothyroidism Type 2

The Epidemic

Mark Starr M.D.

Mark Starr Trust

D0354677

PUBLISHER'S NOTE:

AN IMPORTANT CAUTION TO OUR READERS:

This book is not a medical manual and cannot take the place of personalized medical advice and treatment from a qualified physician. The reader should regularly consult a physician in matters relating to his or her health, particularly with respect to any symptoms that may require diagnosis or treatment. Although certain medical procedures and medical professionals are mentioned in this book, no endorsement, warranty or guarantee by the author is intended. Every attempt has been made to ensure that the information contained in this book is current, however, due to the fact that research is ongoing, some of the material may be invalidated by new findings. The author and publisher cannot guarantee that the information and advice in this book are safe and proper for every reader. For that reason, this book is sold without warranties or guarantees of any kind, expressed or implied, and the author and publisher disclaim any liability, loss or damage caused by the contents. If you do not wish to be bound by these cautions and conditions, you may return your copy to the publisher for a full refund.

Copyright ©2005, 2007, 2009 by Mark Starr Trust

Printed in the United States of America

All rights reserved. No part of this book may be reproduced in any form or by any electronic or mechanical means, including information storage and retrieval systems, without permission in writing from the publisher, except by a reviewer who may quote brief passages in a review.

Starr, Mark
Hypothyroidism Type 2: The Epidemic

ISBN-10:	0-9752624-0-8
ISBN-13:	978-0-9752624-0-5
LCCN:	2004094750
Cover design:	Christy Salinas
Editing:	Thomas D. Boc, B.Sc., D.D.S.

Third printing 2009

Published by
Mark Starr Trust
Columbia, MO
www.type2hypothyroidism.com

Dedication

Ben Starr and Virginia Bliss Starr, my dear parents, made this work possible. My deepest gratitude is extended to Dr. Thomas D. Boc for his excellent advice and considerable time editing the book.

I owe much to my mentors, thank you Hans Kraus M.D., Lawrence S. Sonkin M.D., Ph.D., Andrew A. Fischer M.D., Ph.D., Norman J. Marcus M.D., and William J. Rea M.D. Also, the Broda O. Barnes M.D. Research Foundation has been instrumental in my work on hormones.

For helping edit the final drafts of this book, my thanks to Bruce Clibborn, Tom Loyd, Carol Petersen, Drs. Marcus and Elizabeth Plourde, Dr. Robban Sica, Brenda Wilson, and my dear brother and sister, Steven Starr and Dr. Sydney Starr. Peggy Redfern contributed graphic designs and Gary Kaczmarek enhanced many of the photographs.

TABLE OF CONTENTS

LIST OF TABLES

Those who can't remember the past

are condemned to repeat it.

—George Santayana (1863-1952)

Foreword

You hold in your hands a book, which may well lead you to understanding more about your health and your illnesses than anything that you have ever read. This book is not just about thyroid disorders, but also about the environment in which we live and how that environment may be affecting your entire endocrine or hormone system. As you probably realize, your hormones control every aspect of your life from the ability to raise a family to how well you are able to handle stress without becoming ill or depressed.

This story is really very simple; we are living in an environment where thyroid disease has become an epidemic throughout our society. Unfortunately, this disease is not recognized by most family doctors or even by most specialists. Why? The average physician has virtually stopped physically examining their patients and listening to their medical history, and instead, relies on blood tests to determine their diagnoses. In the area of thyroid disease this approach has proven to be a disaster. The problem with many thyroid and endocrine disorders is that they may occur slowly over several decades. Many of the signs and symptoms of thyroid disease are often attributed to aging. In fact, thyroid disease accelerates the aging process. Most importantly, the thyroid gland is the master control center for the metabolic functions of every single cell in your body. Therefore, a problem with your thyroid gland or with the way thyroid hormones are utilized within the body will produce profound changes in every aspect of your life. Unfortunately, thyroid blood tests do not measure the ability of mitochondria (the small entity within the cell that produces energy) within your cells to use thyroid hormone, nor do they measure the degree to which your thyroid hormone is able to enter the cell to allow normal metabolism. Herein lies the problem with our modern medical approach to understanding thyroid disease.

My own family has been a casualty of this modern approach to caring for patients. I am an Oral and Maxillofacial Surgeon with a background in molecular biology. I have been blessed with two wonderful daughters. From the time of my early childhood I suffered from chronic multiple allergies, chronic respiratory infections and severe hay fever. During the winter, I seemed to catch a cold every other month, and it took weeks for me to recover. During the summer, I also caught colds and took allergy medications continuously. When my daughters, Lauren and Allyson, were born they immediately began the same complex of symptoms and illnesses that I had suffered for more than four decades. Our doctors told us that lots of children have colds, and we should just watch the dust and pollen levels. I was also told to make sure I gave them antibiotics when their colds turned into sinus infections. For many years, that is exactly what I did with numerous trips to the ear, nose, and throat (ENT) specialists to help manage their sinus and respiratory problems.

When I became a little older, another change occurred. I started getting very tired. I would come home after work, eat dinner, and sit on the sofa waiting for 9 PM to come so I could crawl into bed and sleep. I also noticed that I was always feeling cold. When the energy crisis occurred in our nation, I could not understand how anyone could possibly live with their thermostat set at 68 degrees. I complained about these symptoms to my doctor. He ordered multiple laboratory blood tests, including thyroid tests. He found that everything was "normal." I told him to test again, since I was really not feeling well, and his reply was "you are simply aging." This pattern went on for seven years. Each year I would go in for my annual check-up, telling my doctor that my symptoms were getting worse, and each year he would repeat all the blood tests and tell me "you are just getting older." In year eight of this sequence, I diagnosed myself with a thyroid disorder since I now had 11 of the 15 common symptoms of the illness. I told my physician that I really didn't care about his lab results, and I wanted to begin a trial of thyroid hormone. He told me it was not healthy or wise for me to "play" doctor. He reordered my lab tests; the results confirmed his position that I was fine. However, I knew I was NOT fine. By this time I had also gained about 40 lbs. that I could not exercise off due to my chronic fatigue, which seemed to get much worse when I tried to exercise. Clearly, in my view, I was going downhill with no end point in sight. My doctor told me, "Nothing is wrong and you need to accept the fact that a loss of energy is a part of aging and completely normal."

Dr. Mark Starr was referred to my office for evaluation of a bone defect in his lower jaw. We discussed his problem at length and decided on a course of treatment. I asked him what kind of doctor he was, and he told me that his background included sports medicine and hormone disorders. I then asked him if he would listen to my history. On hearing my story, he told me I needed to come to his office for a complete evaluation, and he would try to help me. His approach was completely different. On my first visit to his office, he spent over an hour taking my medical history and the medical history of illness in my entire family. He was interested in the illnesses that my grandparents and parents had encountered. He explained that thyroid illness often has a genetic link. Dr. Starr also repeated the laboratory tests, but he explained that thyroid disease is often missed on lab tests, and my history and symptoms were far more important. He then told me to go home and to start taking my temperature each morning when I woke up and before I got out of bed. I came back the following week, showed him my morning temperatures, and he promptly told me my basal body temperatures were nearly two degrees below normal. He immediately started me on thyroid hormone medication.

Within three months, my fatigue had significantly improved. I noticed that my mental acuity was also much better. My chronic chilly feelings had disappeared. Up to that point, I had never realized that I had always felt cold. A few months later, the feeling of impending doom that I had experienced since childhood disappeared. To my amazement, I was feeling young again. At that point, I brought both of my daughters in for evaluation. They also needed thyroid hormone. Within just a few months, their colds diminished in intensity and duration. Their school attendance markedly improved, and one of my daughters noticed a significant improvement in her grades and academic performance. They both were more active and happy. Needless to say, I was astounded. My family and I were healthier than we had ever been.

I found that my happiness concerning my newfound health was mixed with anger toward the medical profession for the decades of suffering I had endured, for no other reason than my mistaken belief that my doctor knew more about my health than I did. My doctor ignored my symptoms and relied on his laboratory more than his brain to make a diagnosis. There are countless thousands of people who are in failing health because their doctors are not listening to what the patient is trying to tell them about their illnesses. They have been trained to rely on blood tests more than on the history and examination of the patient. Further deepening the problem is the almost universal loss of the family-doctor relationship, which gave the physician a built-in knowledge of the history and course of illnesses that came with the family. Thyroid disease has been well documented for decades, yet most physicians have a difficult time accepting that many of their patients with normal blood tests suffer from hypothyroidism. The literature in medicine is full of the answers doctors need to know; however, these papers go largely unread. Early responders are the small fraction (less than 10%) of the doctors who are able to implement a new idea and put it into practice in their office. So, even if every doctor read all the material concerning thyroid illnesses, only 10% would be ready to act on the knowledge. Since so few doctors have time to read the literature, is there any question why so few are able to diagnose thyroid disease. So what can you do?

The book you are holding in your hands will help you understand the nature and course of thyroid disorders. You will also learn about the chemicals and toxins that prevent normal levels of thyroid hormone in your blood from working properly. The future of your health and the health of your family may depend largely on the story that Dr. Starr has so clearly put forth in this book. You may find that a healthy future is literally being stolen from you by your genes and by the environment. This book will show you a path to restore the health you may have enjoyed as a child.

I hope you enjoy the journey.

Thomas D. Boc, B.Sc., D.D.S.

Introduction

Never in the history of modern medicine has there been an epidemic of such proportion that has gone unrecognized. A well-described and easily treated disease has invaded the vast majority of our homes, wreaking havoc in ways the medical profession could never imagine.

Hypothyroidism is a disease that affects every aspect of our being, from fertility and conception to the grave. The severity and pervasiveness of this illness worsens with each successive generation. Few escape its clutches: heads of state, movie stars, athletes, doctors, blue and white collars alike.

I am a pain specialist. During my long quest for the answer to my own chronic pain, as well as my patients', an unforeseen turn in the road resulted in a mind-boggling conclusion. Hormone problems, chiefly hypothyroidism, not only are responsible for many of our aches and pains but are also responsible for the majority of chronic illnesses found in modern society.

Almost everything addressed in this book was documented many years ago by a number of different doctors. A few attained renowned reputations, while others remain unsung heroes. They were all ahead of their time. Unfortunately, most of their work continues to gather dust in our medical libraries.

Breakthroughs in medicine, particularly changes in perspective, have always been difficult for doctors to accept. The simple concepts of hand washing, sanitation, and the germ theory were scoffed at. Vaccinations were ridiculed, and anesthesia was denigrated for decades. The irrefutable evidence put forth in this book continues to be dismissed, due to the conservative nature of medicine and its entrenched dogma, which is self-perpetuating.

It was my privilege to study with two medical pioneers from the last century, Hans Kraus M.D. and Lawrence Sonkin M.D., Ph.D. Before his retirement, I asked Dr. Sonkin why his research papers on hypothyroidism had not been published in mainstream medical journals. He responded, "Because I sat in the Ivory Tower with the Mavens." Mavens are self-proclaimed experts who, in this instance, use their influence to shape the practice of medicine. Dr. Sonkin's colleagues chose not to publish his research. As is true for the human species in general; money, power, ego, and a large dose of luck profoundly influence our lives and steer the course of medical thinking.

More than one hundred different symptoms may be associated with hypothyroidism. Gradual progression or worsening of symptoms often occurs over many years. This insidious nature of onset, as well as the myriad possible symptoms, has made hypothyroidism difficult for doctors to diagnose. Many decades of progress have been squandered on a plethora of misleading thyroid blood tests. This book will show why these blood tests completely fail to detect Type 2 hypothyroidism.

Problems such as frequent infections, fatigue, anxiety, constipation, skin problems, feeling cold, depression, loss of concentration, menstrual irregularities, obesity, weakness, hypoglycemia, chronic pain, headaches, premature or delayed puberty and menopause, and hyperactivity (ADHD) are only a sampling of possible symptoms. Long-term complications, including heart disease, high blood pressure, stroke, as well as an increased risk of developing cancer, diabetes, dementia, and Alzheimer's are attributable to the epidemic of hypothyroidism. Many more symptoms will be elucidated and discussed.

Today's patients suffering Type 2 hypothyroidism must be treated much more judiciously than those patients from the early twentieth century. Please refer to Chapter 9 (Treatment) prior to initiating hormone therapy.

Proper recognition and treatment of hypothyroidism would prevent much of our illness and suffering. Many millions of lives can be changed for the better and astronomical medical expenses spared if the proposals put forth in this book are accepted.

In submitting this text, the facts, references, and data that will be presented show a convincing picture of an epidemic that has spread across Western Civilization and gone largely unrecognized by the mainstream medical community. Perhaps you will be one of the many people who read this book and take charge of your health by finding a physician who will take the time to listen to your history and examine you clinically to make the diagnosis, instead of making a decision about hypothyroidism based solely on a laboratory test.

This book is a compilation of the overwhelming evidence that not only is the modern laboratory testing used to diagnose hypothyroidism completely inadequate, but the current treatment for the illness is equally lacking in efficacy.

Hypothyroidism Type 2

The Epidemic

Chapter 1
The Thyroid

Endocrine glands produce hormones. Sex hormones are essential for proper development, health, and life itself. For example, the female ovaries make estrogens, progesterone, and some testosterone, and the male testicles manufacture testosterone.

The thyroid gland is butterfly shaped, situated just below the Adam's Apple. The hormones produced from this endocrine gland are responsible for our metabolism.

Frontal View of Thyroid Gland

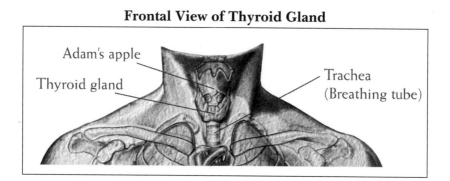

Metabolism is the sum of all physical and chemical processes by which living substances are produced and maintained. Further, metabolism is the transformation by which energy is made available for the uses of the organism. In simple terms, thyroid hormones control the efficiency and speed at which all of our cells work.

Of all your hormones, the thyroid is the most important! Without the crucial influence of thyroid hormones, proper maturation and function of the other hormone glands is not possible.

Thyroid hormones both stimulate the cellular energy production necessary for life, as well as maintain our bodies' relatively constant temperature. The thyroid orchestrates the development of our brain and sexual maturation. Its hormones stimulate synthesis of the protein building blocks that are necessary for normal growth and to replenish the constant turnover of billions of cells that keep us healthy and renew our bodies. Harmful cellular waste products accumulate without proper thyroid function. The immune system is dynamic, energy intensive, and dependent upon normal thyroid function. Susceptibility to infection is one of the hallmarks of hypothyroidism. No matter what you eat or how much you exercise, your health will suffer without proper thyroid function. Appendix A provides a list of the known physiological functions of thyroid hormones.

Do You have Hypothyroidism?

In 1875, Sir William Gull presented the first case reports of hypothyroidism in adults to The Clinical Society of London. By 1888, the symptoms and clinical manifestations of the illness were well described in The Committee of The Clinical Society of London's 200 page report. Most of their findings remain just as true today as they were over a century ago.[1]

Myxedema: The Telltale Sign of Hypothyroidism

In 1878, Dr. William Ord performed an autopsy on a middle-aged woman who succumbed to hypothyroidism. Upon cutting into her skin, he saw tissues that were thickened and boggy. The tissues appeared to be waterlogged, but no water seeped from his incisions. Dr. Ord realized this disease was unique and previously unrecognized.

Dr. Ord summoned a leading chemist named Halleburton to help identify the substance causing the swelling. What they found was an abnormally large accumulation of mucin. Mucin is a normal constituent of our tissues. It is a jelly-like material that spontaneously accumulates in hypothyroidism. Mucin grabs onto water and causes swelling. Dr. Halleburton found 50 times the normal amount of mucin in the woman's skin. Her other tissues also contained excess mucin.

The doctors coined the term "myxedema". "Myx" is the Greek word for mucin and "edema" means swelling. "Myxedema" was adopted as the medical term for hypothyroidism.

The edema or swelling associated with hypothyroidism usually begins around the face, particularly above or below the eyes and along the jaw line. However, the skin on the side of the upper arms may be thickened early in the course of the disease. The swelling associated with hypothyroidism is firm and will eventually spread throughout our body's connective tissues.

One of the many functions of connective tissue is to help hold our bodies' organs and structures together. Connective tissue lines our blood vessels, nervous system, muscles, mucous membranes (such as the sinuses), the gut, as well as each and every cell in our glands and organs. Abnormal accumulation of mucin in these tissues causes swelling and significantly impairs normal function.

This type of swelling is unique to hypothyroidism. Medical textbooks about hypothyroidism state that myxedema is thyroprival (pertaining to or characterized by hypothyroidism) and pathognomonic (specifically distinctive and diagnostic). Translation: if the thickened skin or myxedema is present, you have hypothyroidism.

Do you have myxedema? As I stated, aside from the face, one of the first places affected are the lateral upper arms. Try to pinch the skin as demonstrated in the picture. The swollen skin on this patient's arm, as well as the puffiness in her hand, is a classic demonstration of myxedema.

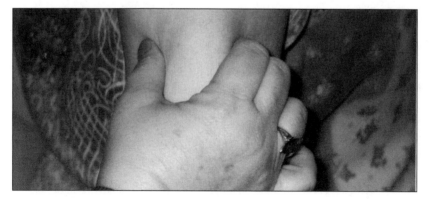

Marked Myxedema

Early twentieth century literature about hypothyroidism included photographs that demonstrated myxedema before and after treatment. The puffiness or myxedema in the patients' faces and hands remarkably improved.[2]

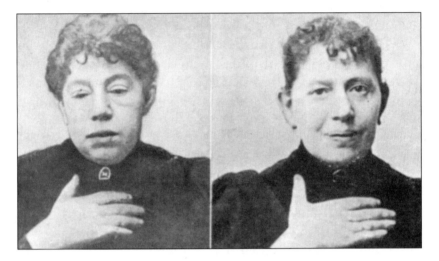

Before treatment   After treatment

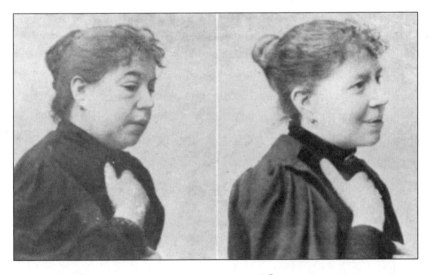

Before treatment   After treatment

Source: Hertoghe, E. *The Practitioner*, Jan 1915, Vol XCIV, No 1, 26-93.

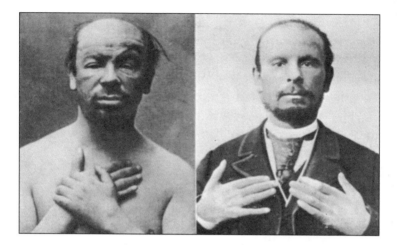

Source: Hertoghe, E. *The Practitioner*, Jan 1915, Vol XCIV, No 1, 26-93.

It is important that you pinch in the same area. Next, try to lift the skin off the underlying tissue on your arm. Normal skin is relatively thin, and you may easily lift it with your thumb and index finger. I have examined a number of patients whose skin is almost impossible to lift. This is due to the marked swelling and glue-like infiltration of mucin in the skin and underlying tissues that result from hypothyroidism. Women's skin usually has slightly more subcutaneous fat than men. Hence, their skin tends to be thicker. There are many different degrees of myxedema. I use *marked, moderate,* and *mild* to describe them. The following picture illustrates normal skin thickness.

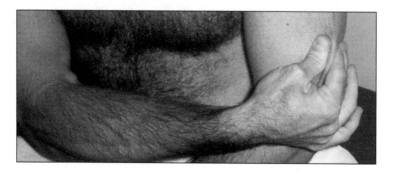

Normal Skin Thickness of the Upper Lateral Arm

Unfortunately, even if your skin is of normal thickness, you may still have the hypothyroidism. It is only one of many signs of this disease.

Today's doctors are not taught to examine for thickened skin or other physical manifestations of the illness. Sophisticated thyroid blood tests are purported to be the sole means for making the diagnosis of hypothyroidism. These tests have replaced the patients' medical histories, complaints, and physical findings upon which the diagnosis was largely based for over half a century before the advent of blood tests.

I raised the ire of many physicians by remarking on the marked myxedema present in their patients. This diagnostic clinical finding has been forgotten, usurped by the almighty thyroid blood tests.

One patient of mine, a 55 year-old suffering from hypothyroidism, returned to his primary care doctor for confirmation of my diagnosis. The patient was obese, suffering chronic pain, fatigue, dry skin, high blood pressure, a slightly irregular heartbeat, and sleep apnea. The skin on his upper arms and the front of his thighs was quite thickened with myxedema. The primary care doctor told the patient the thickened skin was due to his obesity. The patient and his wife were concerned with the conflicting views. Fortunately, he finally decided to follow my advice.

After many months of treatment for hypothyroidism, his chronic fatigue vastly improved, his heartbeat normalized, high blood pressure resolved, and the thickness of his skin normalized. The myxedema had disappeared. I told the patient to tell his primary care doctor that his skin had been on a crash diet. Pictures of his skin one year after beginning thyroid hormones are shown on the next page.

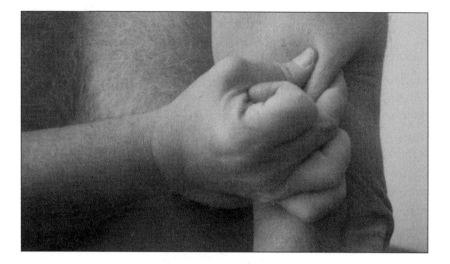

Sleep apnea is also listed in medical texts among the symptoms resulting from hypothyroidism. The 55 year-old patient's sleep apnea has not been resolved, as it is much easier to prevent chronic illnesses than to treat them.

Another patient, when informed of the diagnosis of hypothyroidism, became belligerent and stated, "I'm in perfect condition." I managed to quell the urge to ask what he was doing in my pain clinic if he were so perfect (he suffered from chronic foot pain). The patient returned to work and proceeded to pinch the skin of many co-workers. He refused to accept my diagnosis, during his next visit, because "everybody where I work has thick skin." I'm afraid he was probably correct. The disease is epidemic.

As I noted before, having skin of normal thickness and composition does not exclude the diagnosis of hypothyroidism. A study published in 1955 compared skin biopsies of 26 children with definite hypothyroidism. Only 15 had positive skin biopsy findings of increased mucin.[3] Remember, mucin is a normal constituent of our tissues, and its accumulation is often increased with hypothyroidism. However, the accumulation of mucin may only affect the internal organs and tissues and spare the skin. In other words, you may have hypothyroidism despite having normal skin.

Basal Metabolic Rate

For the first quarter century following the discovery of hypothyroidism, patients' medical histories, symptoms, and physical findings, combined with doctors' awareness, were the only means for making the diagnosis. A trial of thyroid hormones, leading to the resolution of a patient's symptoms and physical manifestations, was confirmation of a correct diagnosis.

In the early twentieth century, a test measuring basal metabolism (the basal metabolic rate or BMR) was developed to aid doctors with the often obscure and difficult diagnosis of hypothyroidism. Just as it sounds, the test measured a person's metabolism by monitoring oxygen consumption for a given height, age, weight, and sex. Normal values were determined for a large number of apparently healthy people.

Hypothyroidism causes our metabolism to slow down. The tiny energy factories called "mitochondria" inside each of our cells do not function properly, because sufficient supplies of chemical energy are lacking. This lowered rate of metabolism was often reflected by the basal metabolism test. However, in order for the BMR test to be accurate, the patient must be free from stress and nervous tension. Nervous tension may result from chronic pain, neuroses, or other problems often associated with hypothyroidism.

Patients were tested after a good night sleep. They were instructed to fast after their evening meal and to travel immediately to the test upon awakening. If they lived too far away, they were hospitalized overnight in an attempt to ensure accuracy.

Basal metabolism tests formerly required a tight clip to be placed on the patient's nose to restrict air flow and a breathing tube inserted in the patient's mouth to measure oxygen consumption. This alone was enough to cause tension, consternation, and confuse the test results. Stressors and tension often resulted in a normal or above average BMR result despite the fact that a patient's metabolism was actually low. A British study tested 100 patients with definite hypothyroidism in 1960. The basal metabolism test confirmed the illness in only 77 of the patients.[4]

A host of brilliant doctors' voices are now silent. Most of their protestations regarding the accuracy of thyroid blood tests have long been forgotten. These doctors successfully treated the illness for decades prior to the advent of thyroid blood tests. Lawrence S. Sonkin M.D., Ph.D. was a twentieth century pioneer in the field of endocrinology. He devoted his long career to research, teaching, and treating thousands of patients at New York Hospital–Cornell Medical Center. Dr. Sonkin referred to hypothyroidism that was not detected by modern blood tests as "Symptomatic Low Metabolism". These patients' thyroid blood tests showed normal function of the thyroid gland. However, the patients manifested obvious clinical symptoms of hypothyroidism and physical findings such as myxedema. Most importantly, they improved when given thyroid hormones. Dr. Sonkin believed their problem was at the cellular level where thyroid hormones perform their tasks.

Dr. Sonkin utilized basal metabolism tests in his research articles to demonstrate the erroneous nature of the supposedly diagnostic blood tests. He knew the basal metabolism tests were fallible as well.[5,6] Dr. Sonkin and other doctors, aware of the test's limitations, advocated trials of thyroid hormones for patients who suffered symptoms and physical characteristics consistent with the disease. **Improvement of patients' symptoms with treatment has always been and will remain the final judge of whether or not a patient needs thyroid hormones.**

The following graph illustrates how many of Dr. Sonkin's patients with normal blood tests responded well to thyroid hormones. One hundred consecutive patients with symptoms of hypothyroidism were tested. The change in basal metabolism and cholesterol levels are plotted on the graph. The darkened circles indicate improvement of symptoms associated with hypothyroidism.[6]

Therapeutic Trials (TSH and/or T-4 normal)

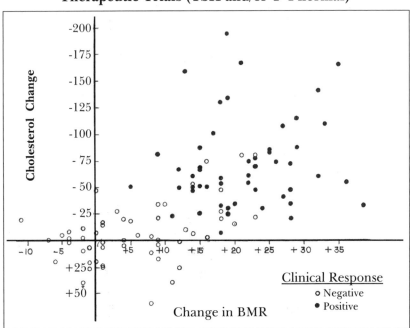

Source: Gelb, H. *Clinical Management of Head, Neck, and TMJ Pain and Dysfunction.*
Philadelphia: W. B. Saunders, 1977. p. 162. Reprinted with permission.

The horizontal line represents the change in basal metabolism (BMR) after a trial of thyroid hormones. Two-thirds (66/100) of the patients' BMRs increased from 10% to 35%. The vertical line represents the drop in patients' cholesterol. After thyroid therapy, over half of the patients' total cholesterol dropped 25 points to 200 points. The solid circles reflect improvement in the symptoms associated with hypothyroidism, indicating that a majority of these patients improved.

During the first half of the twentieth century, prior to complete reliance on blood tests to diagnose hypothyroidism, elevated cholesterol was considered one of the hallmarks of hypothyroidism. Today, increased cholesterol is often mistakenly related to a high fat diet and an indication for expensive cholesterol lowering drugs. (A more detailed discussion on thyroid hormones' influence on cholesterol follows in Chapter 8.)

My Patients' Basal Metabolism and Thyroid Blood Tests

In 1998, I recruited a Ph.D. exercise physiologist to perform basal metabolic rate testing for my pain patients. The doctor was very conscientious and tried to make certain the patients were relaxed and proper procedures followed. He performed basal metabolism tests on 50 consecutive pain patients. **All of these patients had normal thyroid blood tests.**

My 50 patients' metabolism averaged 15% below normal. A significant number of their metabolic rates were in the 30 - 40% below-normal range. Several tests were above average as well. When a basal metabolism test was previously used to aid doctors in making the diagnosis of hypothyroidism, a test result of 10% less than normal or lower was considered strongly indicative of the illness.

I sent copies of the low basal metabolic tests to the patients' primary care physicians along with my diagnosis of hypo-thyroidism. Almost without exception, the test results as well as the patients' textbook symptomatology were ignored. Their physicians simply felt that the blood tests could not be wrong.

An unfortunate 80 year-old woman held the record low metabolism for all my patients. She initially was unable to stay awake during her office visits and summoned all her energy to travel to and from my office. The patient stated she slept for most of the previous 10 years after a new doctor stopped her thyroid medication. He said her blood tests showed she no longer needed thyroid hormones. Despite the fact she had taken the medicine for over 40 years and was doing quite well, the thyroid hormones were stopped. Her basal metabolism test showed a 48% below normal result. I stated that if she was an optimist, she was half alive, and if she was a pessimist, half dead. She felt much better after beginning thyroid. Unfortunately, she returned to her primary care doctor, then did poorly again.

The following pictures are illustrative of the profound effect thyroid hormones have when properly administered. This 34 year-old woman's BMR was minus 39% when the first picture was taken. After only nine months of treatment with desiccated thyroid hormones, there was a remarkable change in her appearance. Her BMR had increased to plus 2%.

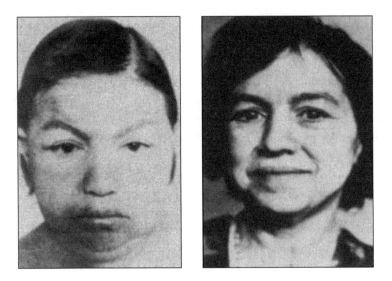

Before treatment   After treatment

Source: Lisser, H., and Escamilla, R. F. *Atlas of Clinical Endocrinology: Including Text of Diagnosis and Treatment*. C.V. Mosby Company, 1957. Reprinted with Permission.

I lost count of how many elderly pain patients related similar stories. Every time their former doctor retired, or they moved, their dosage of thyroid was decreased, changed to the "new type" of synthetic thyroid hormone, or discontinued altogether. The decline of these senior citizens' health almost always began shortly thereafter. None of the prior doctors made the connection between their declining health and the decreased dosage of thyroid hormones. They continued in the belief that the thyroid blood tests could not be wrong.

Basal Temperature

An extremely prevalent symptom of hypothyroidism is a lowering of body temperature. The low temperature is a direct reflection of decreased metabolism. Hypothyroidism is not the only problem that may lower the patients' temperature, but it is definitely the most common.

The 200-page report on hypothyroidism by The Clinical Society of London in 1888 was the most comprehensive description of the illness for its time. Their findings concluded that patients' temperatures were almost always subnormal, "although it may now and then rise to the normal standard or even a degree or two higher".[1]

Dr. Ord, the renowned British doctor who named the illness in 1877, contributed a chapter entitled "Myxedema" to a landmark medical text published in 1901. Under the section concerning symptoms, Dr. Ord stated, "The temperature of the body is generally below normal, 97 or 96 degrees Fahrenheit (°F) being a common record; and the patients are extremely sensitive to cold."[7]

The first description of the milder forms of hypothyroidism was published in a 1915 medical journal entitled *The Practitioner*. The author, Dr. Eugene Hertoghe, stated, "Hypothermia [low temperature] is an almost invariable accompaniment of even the slighter forms of thyroid insufficiency. Such patients, the younger ones more particularly, complain of chilliness of the hands and feet; they never feel warm, even in bed."[2]

One of the twentieth century's most prolific researchers with regard to hypothyroidism was Broda O. Barnes M.D., Ph.D. The Broda O. Barnes M.D. Research Foundation was established as a nonprofit research foundation dedicated to the dissemination of his work as well as other medical pioneers in the field of endocrinology (the study of hormones). Dr. Barnes received a master's degree in biochemistry at Case Western Reserve University in 1930, followed by a physiology Ph.D. from the University of Chicago in 1931. His mentor was Professor A.J. Carlson, one of America's pioneers in the field of physiology. Dr. Carlson assigned Broda Barnes to study the physiology of the thyroid gland for his doctorate. At the time, in 1931, the understanding of complex hormone functions such as the thyroid was in its early stages.

Dr. Barnes continued thyroid research while teaching endocrinology for the next five years at the University of Chicago before obtaining his medical degree from Rush Medical College in 1937. The rest of his life was devoted to treating patients and doing clinical and scientific research with regard to thyroid-related illnesses. Dr. Barnes died in 1988 at the age of 82.

Dr. Barnes practiced endocrinology before the advent of thyroid blood tests. He always measured patients' temperatures just prior to running their BMR. His research confirmed the presence of subnormal temperatures in both animals and humans suffering hypothyroidism. Thyroid hormones raised temperatures. If too much thyroid was given, the temperatures often climbed above normal.

By the beginning of the twentieth century, doctors had already established the fact that patients suffering from hyperthyroidism, the overproduction of thyroid hormones, demonstrated above normal temperatures (hyperthyroidism is the medical term for the opposite of hypothyroidism). Dr. Barnes and other prominent doctors also mentioned the abnormal elevation of body temperature, "pyrexia," if too much thyroid hormone was administered to a hypothyroid patient.[4,7,8]

Dr. Barnes' paper, "Basal Temperature vs. Basal Metabolism," was published in "The Journal of the American Medical Association" in 1942. In this study of 1,000 patients with low basal metabolism tests and symptoms of hypothyroidism, all had subnormal temperatures (unless an infection was present). Without exception, thyroid therapy led to an elevation of their temperatures. Dr. Barnes stated, "Very few patients with subnormal temperature fail to respond to thyroid therapy, both as to relief of symptoms and to elevation of temperatures."[9] In addition, he presented case studies of patients that demonstrated problems associated with the BMR testing, which could be avoided if the patients' basal temperatures were used in its place.

Several patients appeared to have overactive thyroid function or hyperthyroidism. These patients exhibited symptoms such as tremor, rapid heart rates, anxiety, and elevated BMRs. Prior doctors had already made the diagnosis of hyperthyroidism in several of these patients. Dr. Barnes examined these patients and measured their basal temperatures. Despite having elevated BMRs and symptoms consistent with hyperthyroidism, he found their temperatures to be low. His diagnosis of hypothyroidism, the exact opposite of the other doctors, was confirmed when the patients' symptoms resolved after treatment with thyroid hormones.

This illustrates one of the most confounding and problematic aspects about the diagnosis of hypothyroidism: the fact that it may produce completely opposite symptoms in affected patients. Many patients tend to be overweight, sluggish, have slow heart rates, and low BMRs. A minority of the patients with hypothyroidism may be underweight, have rapid heart rates, and suffer tremors, anxiety, and increased BMRs. The latter may be due to the nervous tension that often results from inadequate thyroid stimulus. My teacher, Dr. Sonkin, used the analogy that such patients were running on watered-down gasoline. They are constantly trying to compensate for their inadequate energy supplies by running in overdrive and are unable to relax. In an attempt to compensate for low thyroid function, the body may produce excess adrenaline (the fight or flight hormone) and other adrenal hormones as a response to stress. This nervous tension may cause tremor, anxiety, and falsely elevated BMRs. However, these symptoms are commonly attributed to <u>hyper</u>thyroidism. In 1973, Dr. Barnes stated that even after 35 years of practicing medicine, he occasionally could not differentiate between <u>hyper</u>thyroidism and hypothyroidism without using the thermometer.[10]

For example, a 22 year-old woman had been nervous and underweight for years. She had a fine tremor in her hands, and her heart rate was elevated to 110 beats per minute. The BMR was plus 18% when tested at a prior university and plus 8% when tested by Dr. Barnes. However, her basal temperature was subnormal. Her hypothyroid state was confirmed when her heart rate normalized, her tremor improved, and she gained weight with thyroid hormone treatment.[9,10]

After treatment, the patients who initially had elevated BMRs and subnormal temperatures had normal BMRs. Administration of thyroid hormones is not supposed to decrease the BMR. In fact, it is supposed to do just the opposite. So, why did administering thyroid hormones allow normalization of basal metabolism? This occurred because the nervous tension and excess adrenal output were eliminated. I have witnessed numerous such cases including my own. My constant foot tapping, chronic teeth clenching, and inability to relax were beyond my control. After supplying what my body so desperately needed, thyroid hormones, those problems are now distant memories.

Normal Body Temperatures

During a tour of duty in World War II, Dr. Barnes studied 1,000 soldiers' basal temperatures. Armed with thermometers, he would head for the soldiers' barracks before reveille. One thermometer would be placed in their mouth, one in their armpit (axilla), and one in their rectum. If no sign of upper respiratory infection was present, he found that the oral temperature was within one-tenth degree of the axilla (armpit), and the rectal temperature was eight-tenths higher. Dr. Barnes also studied more than 1,000 additional patients' oral and axillary temperatures before the publication of these findings in his article, "Basal Temperature versus Basal Metabolism."[9,10] These findings conflict with standard medical texts that state the axillary temperature is one degree lower than the oral temperature and two degrees below the rectal temperature. However, no references for these conclusions were cited in the medical textbooks I checked. Dr. Barnes found that oral temperatures were elevated more than axillary temperatures in patients that had chronic sinusitis or upper respiratory infections. Since these ailments are extremely common, they may explain why the medical literature conflicts with Dr. Barnes' research.

Taking Your Basal Temperature

Just like the BMR, the basal temperature should be taken after a good night rest with no food, exercise, nor excitement for 12 hours. Many patients who are hypothyroid may cover themselves with an excess number of blankets or quilts, sleep on a heated waterbed, or wear long underwear, socks, or layers of clothes to bed. All of these measures will falsely elevate the basal temperature.

Dr. Barnes recommended mercury thermometers for basal temperature tests. However, mercury thermometers are no longer available. New alcohol glass thermometers are a good second choice. Digital thermometer readings may fluctuate several tenths of a degree during consecutive readings, so they are a poor third choice.

To test your basal temperature, the thermometer is placed snugly in the armpit for 10 minutes before arising in the morning. Temperature readings of 97.8 to 98.2 °F (36.6 to 36.8 °C) are considered normal. Readings below 97.8 °F are highly indicative of hypothyroidism.

Remember: This is your final reading. Do not add one degree to compensate for it not being an oral reading.

Several days of basal temperature measurements are recommended. Men can perform the test on any day when they are not rushed. Women's temperatures fluctuate during their menstrual cycle, and their tests should be taken on the second and third days after menstrual flow starts. After menopause or before puberty, women's basal temperature may be taken on any day.

Small children may be checked by rectal temperature for two minutes. The rectal temperature is normally eight-tenths to one degree higher than the armpit. Therefore, 98.6 to 99.2 °F would be considered normal.

Dr. Barnes did not recommend oral temperatures for basal temperature testing, because there is a high frequency of chronic, low-grade sinus and upper respiratory tract infections associated with hypothyroidism. These infections, or chronic sinusitis, and post nasal drip will spuriously elevate one's oral temperature. Severe arthritis, pain, hyperthyroidism, and other less common problems may also elevate the basal temperature.

Potential Symptoms of Hypothyroidism; from the Broda O. Barnes M.D. Research Foundation list:

Fatigue
Decreased sex drive
Candida (yeast infections)
Dry skin
Premature aging
Infertility
Constipation
P.M.S.
Repeated infections
Headaches
Hypertension
   (i.e., high blood
   pressure)
Brittle nails
Birth defects
Mental disorders
Endometriosis
Diabetes
Multiple sclerosis (MS)
Memory impairment
Cancer
Nervousness
Heart attack/stroke
Hair loss
High cholesterol
Intolerance to heat
Nutritional imbalances

Muscle weakness
Low immune system
Overweight
Arthritis/gout
Low blood pressure
Depression
Osteoporosis
Joint/muscle pain
Heart palpitations
Cystic breasts/ovaries
Chronic fatigue
Intolerance to cold
Hyperinsulinemia

Source: Broda O. Barnes M.D. Research Foundation at: www.brodabarnes.org/

This is only a partial list. One glaring omission is menstrual disorders. A whole chapter was devoted to this topic in Dr. Barnes' book, *Hypothyroidism, the Unsuspected Illness*.[4]

Below is a list of symptoms and signs from a recent, prominent, medical textbook. A detailed discussion of symptoms associated with hypothyroidism follows in Chapter 8.

<u>Symptoms</u>

Fatigue
Lethargy
Sleepiness
Mental impairment
Depression
Cold intolerance
Hoarseness
Dry skin
Decreased perspiration
Weight gain
Decreased appetite
Constipation
Menstrual disturbances
Arthralgia (pain in a joint)
Paresthesia (abnormal sensations such as burning, prickling, or feeling as if tiny insects are crawling on your skin)

<u>Signs</u>

Slow movements
Slow speech
Hoarseness
Bradycardia (slow heart rate)
Dry skin
Nonpitting edema (myxedema)
Hyporeflexia (diminished reflexes)
Delayed relaxation of reflexes

Source: Braverman, L. E., and Utiger, R. D. *Warner & Ingbar's The Thyroid: A Fundamental and Clinical Text.* 8th ed. New York: Lippincott Williams & Wilkins Publishers, 2000. Reprinted with permission.

By the end of 1998, I began to realize the profound prevalence of hypothyroidism. In fact, I began to believe a majority of Americans were suffering from the illness. How could I possibly arrive at such an astonishing conclusion? The answer follows.

Hypothyroid Mother with Cretin Child

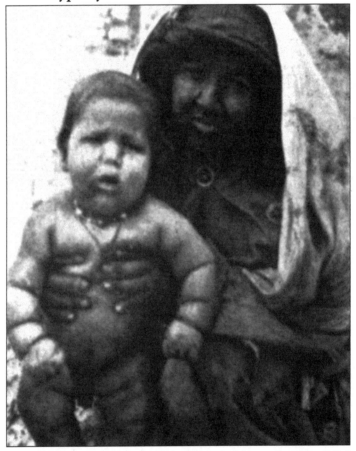

Hypothyroid mother and 2 year-old cretinous child (severe hypothyroidism), note myxedema puffiness of child's body, thick flat nose, open mouth, and narrow eye slits.

Source: Lisser, H., and Escamilla, R. F. *Atlas of Clinical Endocrinology: Including Text of Diagnosis and Treatment*. C.V. Mosby Company, 1957. Reprinted with Permission.

Chapter 2
Unrecognized Giants of Medicine

After I suffered a low back injury in high school, 20 years of intermittent back pain ensued. Doctors, who specialize in physical medicine and rehabilitation, such as I, are trained in the conservative (nonsurgical) treatment of pain. Nevertheless, despite daily exercise, physical therapy, and chiropractic treatments, my back pain persisted. Many of my patients followed this same discouraging pattern of chronic pain.

In 1994, following medical school and residency training, I moved to New York City in order to study with (and be treated by) several great medical pioneers from the twentieth century.

Andrew A. Fischer M.D., Ph.D. was chairman of the Department of Physical Medicine and Rehabilitation at the Bronx New York Veterans Hospital. Dr. Fischer emigrated from Czechoslovakia in 1968 before the Soviet invasion. He was already a physician, as well as a Ph.D., when he began his residency training in Physical Medicine and Rehabilitation at New York University's famous Rusk Institute of Rehabilitation Medicine. Renowned in the treatment of soft tissue injuries (muscles, ligaments, tendons), Dr. Fischer published scores of articles on the subject. I saw him lecture at a national conference the previous year and was invited to study with him.

During my stay, Dr. Fischer introduced me to Hans Kraus M.D. who was an associate professor of Physical Medicine and Rehabilitation at the Rusk Institute during Dr. Fischer's training. Despite being in his late 80s, Dr. Kraus continued to work at the New York Pain Treatment Program at Lenox Hill Hospital, where he worked with Norman Marcus M.D. who later became President of the American Academy of Pain Medicine.

One of the highlights of my life was having the opportunity to study with Dr. Kraus. Both he and Dr. Marcus treated and tutored me regarding Kraus's techniques. Dr. Kraus trained a team of physical therapists whom I was also fortunate to study with and be treated by.

Dr. Kraus, an orthopedic surgeon trained in Vienna, developed the treatment for one of the largest organ systems in our body, the muscles. He never operated again after elucidating the proper treatment of muscles and ligaments. In 1954, he published a landmark report that astonishingly revealed that 50% of American children failed to pass a basic test of postural trunk strength and flexibility, when only 4% of their European counterparts failed. President Eisenhower began The President's Council on Physical Fitness after discussing the health of American children with Dr. Kraus.[12,13]

Dr. Kraus and Sonya Webber Ph.D. developed The *Y's Way to a Healthy Back* exercise program for chronic back pain, which was published by Alexander Melleby.[72] Over 300,000 chronic back pain sufferers participated. A study that involved 11,000 program participants revealed 80% of the participants reported significant or complete relief of pain.[14,72,94]

Dr. Kraus worked with President Kennedy's endocrinologist, Eugene Cohen M.D. (JFK had hypothyroidism and Addison's disease). Dr. Kraus was teaching at NYU's Rusk Rehabilitation Center while Dr. Cohen was Professor of Medicine at the New York Hospital–Cornell Medical Center, providing them with the opportunity to collaborate in the treatment of pain patients. Dr. Cohen believed Dr. Kraus was one of the great medical pioneers of the twentieth century and insisted that he be summoned to treat Kennedy's back after all others failed. JFK's lower back pain was relieved by Kraus's treatment after three prior orthopedic surgeries had failed. JFK had planned to establish a national institute devoted to the study and treatment of muscles.[14] Kennedy's assassination dramatically altered the course of modern medicine and its approach to chronic pain. I recommend all of Dr. Kraus' books including his biography, *Into The Unknown*, by Susan Schwartz.

Dr. Kraus continued to work with Dr. Cohen as well as one of his colleagues, Lawrence Sonkin M.D., Ph.D., another endocrinologist from the New York Hospital–Cornell Medical

Center in New York City. These three physicians worked together for the remainder of their combined careers. In his published works, Dr. Kraus included a chapter written by Dr. Sonkin regarding hormonal imbalance and its relationship to pain.

It was my great fortune to have been the last student of both Drs. Kraus and Sonkin. Dr. Kraus continued to consult at the New York Pain Treatment Program at Lenox Hill Hospital until three months prior to his death in March 1996. Dr. Sonkin retired shortly thereafter and died in January 2002.

I intended to study in New York for six weeks before returning to the Midwest to begin employment. However, I was seeing patients who were recuperating from many of their aches and pains by treatment methods I had previously never witnessed. Six weeks turned into six months, which turned into two years before I was satisfied with my additional training.

The Bronx V. A. Hospital offered an unlimited supply of pain patients. I spent over a year devoted to their treatment. Many patients made significant or complete recoveries using treatment techniques for muscle pain. However, my own pain, as well as that of a large number of the patients' remained problematic.

The tremendous significance of muscle pain is largely neglected by our teaching institutions. Muscles comprise almost half our bodies and are full of nerves. The subject of pain will be discussed in more detail in Chapter 8.

Prior to moving to New York, I suspected that I was suffering from hypothyroidism. My mother and brother were already taking medication for the illness, and my grandmother had also been diagnosed just prior to her death. I was cold most of the time, had dry skin and hair, sore muscles, was losing my ability to concentrate, and becoming more and more fatigued. The doctors at the University Hospital where I trained assured me that I could not possibly have hypothyroidism, because my blood tests were normal. Fortunately, I chose to go to New York and found the answers I had been seeking. Dr. Sonkin confirmed my diagnosis of hypothyroidism after the initial questioning and physical examination. A slowly increasing dose of thyroid hormone, as well as treatments for my muscles using Dr. Kraus's techniques, began to relieve most of my physical complaints, including the pain.

Returning from New York to my home in Missouri in 1996, I was brimming with enthusiasm and ready to tackle the most difficult pain patients. During the next two years in private practice, the overwhelming pervasiveness of hypothyroidism gradually unfolded. Many patients either did not respond or only partially responded to my treatments. The more I suspected hypothyroidism, the more I studied the disease, and the more I looked, the more I found. Dr. Sonkin forewarned me about the high prevalence of hormone problems, especially hypothyroidism, found in chronic pain patients. By 1998, it appeared to me that the vast majority of all chronic pain patients were hypothyroid. It was more than a little daunting to think I was the only person who knew and understood the magnitude of the problem.

One of America's greatest doctors, William Osler M.D., helped put Johns Hopkins Hospital on the map in the late nineteenth century. Dr. Osler taught the importance of listening to patients. He would say, "If you give the patient enough time, they will make the diagnosis for you." He also stressed how imperative it is that the doctor knows what questions to ask and what physical findings to look for. He stated this as, "The eye can not see what the mind does not know." Emulating Dr. Kraus's techniques meant spending many hours talking, examining, and touching the patients, which culminated in my astounding conclusion:

Most chronic pain is just one symptom of a much greater problem, which accounts for the majority of patients' illnesses. The problem is hypothyroidism.

On their initial examination, many of my patients' complaints and physical findings (consistent with hypothyroidism) would be listed in their patient summary. A typical list for one of my chronic pain patients might read:

Patient has a history of dry skin, fatigue, menorrhagia (heavy periods), chronic sinusitis, TMJ with persistent teeth clenching, insomnia, chronic pain, as well as a positive family history for hypothyroidism, hypertension (high blood pressure), diabetes, heart disease, allergies, and cancer.

Regarding the physical exam: "The patient has moderate myxedema over the proximal upper and lower extremities with very dry skin that is tender to the pinch. Her hands and feet are cool and clammy to the touch, nails yellowed and ridged, dry hair, lateral thinning of the eyebrows, delayed ankle reflexes, as well as diffuse tender points and trigger points throughout her muscles."

This patient already had a hysterectomy, gallbladder surgery, and two C-sections. Her basal temperature was later found to be about 97.0 °F. A list of symptoms such as these was the rule rather than the exception among my chronic pain patients.

I traveled to San Diego in 1998 in order to become board certified in pain medicine. Several days of review courses regarding the latest research on pain treatment were followed by a two-day national conference for doctors who were all pain specialists. One lecture was devoted to the treatment of muscle pain. However, there was no mention or lectures regarding hormone imbalances. Chronic pain is almost always attributed to arthritis, pinched nerves, mental disorders, tendonitis, or nebulous pain syndromes such as fibromyalgia.

In the spring of 1999, a colleague of mine picked up a used book as a gift for me. He knew of my keen interest in hypothyroidism. The book was Dr. Barnes' *Hypothyroidism, The Unsuspected Illness*. Here was confirmation of all I suspected and much more. I felt elated. My office manager and I went out to celebrate the discovery of Dr. Barnes and the Barnes Foundation, which continues to distribute his work. I admitted great relief that others were also aware of the silent epidemic, while at the same time, I felt a slight disappointment for not having been the first to recognize the magnitude of the problem. Dr. Barnes referred to himself as a "Johnny come lately". Almost every time he discovered a new benefit from thyroid therapy, his research uncovered a previous article on the same subject. Most of those articles are listed in the bibliographies of his books. Mainstream medicine never recognized the profound importance of these studies. Perhaps the treatment was just too simple for the average physician's complex perspectives on disease management.

Case Study

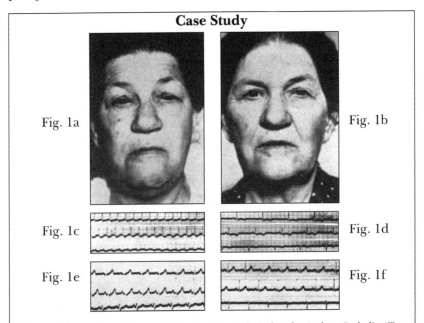

Fig. 1a   Fig. 1b

Fig. 1c   Fig. 1d

Fig. 1e   Fig. 1f

Source: Lisser, H., and Escamilla, R. F. *Atlas of Clinical Endocrinology: Including Text of Diagnosis and Treatment.* C.V. Mosby Company, 1957. Reprinted with Permission.

Figure 1a. Myxedema in woman, aged 51 years. Presenting complaint: attacks of palpitation and rapid heart action for previous 17 years. Note myxedematous puffiness of face, especially under eyes, and narrow palpebral apertures, giving sleepy appearance; voice tones were hollow, rasping and leathery; rarely perspired; feet felt "frozen"; appetite poor; constipated. BMR,-31%.

Figure 1b. Same patient's appearance after 1 month on thyroid; note striking change, loss of myxedematous puffiness and return of bright alert expression. BMR now -10%. Speech, movements and cerebration much livelier.

Figure 1c. Electrocardiogram during attack, before treatment: typical paroxysmalnodal tachycardia; rate 168; depressed S-T intervals; flattened T waves.

Figure 1d. Electrocardiogram 6 days later, before treatment: bradycardia, rate 40; inversion of T waves in all 3 leads.

Figure 1e. Electrocardiogram after 6 months treatment with thyroid alone. Note striking improvement; rate now normal (79), T waves upright in all leads. No further attacks of paroxysmal tachycardia [rapid heart beat].

Figure 1f. Electrocardiogram after 21 months treatment: rate 72; T waves still upright. Thyroid dose, 1 to 1 1/2 grains (0.065 to 0.1 Gm.) daily.

Chapter 3
Heart Attacks: The Graz Autopsy Studies

Broda O. Barnes M.D., Ph.D. made a serendipitous discovery about the effects of hypothyroidism through the American Medical Society of Vienna. Empress Maria Theresa, renowned eighteenth century Austrian monarch, passed a law that mandated autopsies be performed on all hospital deaths occurring in Austria's second largest city, Graz. The city lay in the heart of an area that suffered endemic hypothyroidism and goiters. The primitive state of medicine in Graz during the eighteenth century prompted the Empress to enact the law. At that time, 98 out of 100 newborns were dying in Graz. From that time forth, the pathologists in Graz performed the autopsies. About 75% of the total deaths were autopsied each year, more than enough to establish any changes in the patterns of death.

The Empress could not have imagined that her law would help solve so many of the great medical questions of the twentieth century.[10] The beginnings of modern medicine are traced directly to autopsy studies. In the early eighteenth century, doctors began to correlate clinical symptoms and physical examination with post-mortem findings at autopsy.

Autopsy developed into an essential routine at the great medical centers. Only then did medicine slowly emerge from the archaic belief in humoralism, put forth over 14 centuries earlier. Prior to this change in medical practice, humoralism was the ancient theory that health and illness resulted from a balance or imbalance of bodily liquids (humors). One of the most common treatments associated with this practice was bloodletting. This medieval belief relentlessly persisted into the early nineteenth century. For example, in 1827, 33 million leeches were imported into France.[15]

Autopsy became and has remained the "Gold Standard" for evaluating the presence and extent of disease. Repeated studies, covering the last 50 years, showed the frequency of diagnostic errors made by patients' doctors to be between 40% and 50%. This includes 10% misdiagnoses (the primary cause of death was wrong), 10% false-positives (the doctors assigned a problem that did not exist), and 20% to 30% false-negative diagnoses (the doctors missed an additional diagnosis).[16] Even today, with increasingly sophisticated medical tools, such as MRI, the percentages of diagnostic errors made by doctors remains unchanged.[70]

Much of the credit for creating the science of medicine is given to Rudolph Virchow M.D. (1821-1902). So much so, it earned him the title: Father of Pathology. Dr. Virchow was the first to realize that the basis for disease involved the cell. His revelations included: cells are derived only from other cells, and diseased structures are a variation or disturbance of the normal cells and structures. The melding of cellular science, microbiology, physiology, and pathology finally had taken place. Dr. Virchow's teachings put an end to humoralism. His Berlin headquarters became the world's foremost medical center during the second half of the nineteenth century.

Dr. Virchow was also the first to describe the changes that occur during the process of hardening of the arteries. The first change or "lesion" in an artery on the road to atherosclerosis is inflammation. "Inflammation is a localized protective response caused by injury or destruction of tissues, which serves to destroy, dilute, or wall off (sequester) both the injurious agent and the injured tissue."[17] These cellular changes are reviewed, in an article from *The New England Journal of Medicine* (1999) entitled, "Atherosclerosis-An Inflammatory Disease". It states, "In fact, the earliest type of lesion, the so-called fatty streak, which is common in infants and young children, is a pure inflammatory lesion."[17]

In general, most infections have some degree of systemic effect, which may involve our arteries. Infection fighting cells course through the arteries. However, the underlying cause of the inflammatory response in the arteries that leads to atherosclerosis continues to be debated. Dr. Barnes believed the recurrent infections associated with hypothyroidism to be largely responsible. He cited autopsy studies from 1969 that showed evidence of atherosclerosis in all of the children by age three, whether they were from third world countries or modernized nations.[18]

Dr. Virchow stated near the end of his career, "If I could live my life over again, I would devote it to proving that germs seek their natural habitat—diseased tissue—rather than being the cause of the disease; e.g., mosquitoes seek the stagnant water, but do not cause the pool to become stagnant." The father of modern medicine correctly surmised that those who were susceptible to infection had an underlying physiological problem that predisposed them to their illness. In the vast majority of the population, that problem is hypothyroidism.

The association between damaged arteries and hypothyroidism was first noted in an 1877 autopsy by Dr. William M. Ord and was firmly established by The 1888 Clinical Society of London's report.[1,19] A flurry of research followed the 1888 report. Viennese doctors as well as a London physiologist, Dr. Victor Horsley, began removing thyroid glands from animals to study the consequences. Greatly accelerated atherosclerosis (hardening of the arteries) occurred after removal of thyroid glands in all of the animals. They found that administering thyroid hormones to these animals halted the progression of atherosclerosis.

At the University of Chicago in the 1930s, Dr. Barnes removed the thyroid glands of baby rabbits to demonstrate to his students the physiological changes of hypothyroidism. The rabbits' life spans were halved. Most of the physical changes associated with hypothyroidism, including recurrent infections and markedly accelerated arterial damage, were demonstrable. However, the mental changes were not.

Dr. Barnes believed hypothyroidism was the underlying cause of the tremendous increase in heart attacks during the twentieth century. Heart attacks were extremely rare among his large group of patients being treated for hypothyroidism. Yet, they were increasing dramatically in the general populace.

Dr. Barnes hoped to find the answers from the Graz autopsies. Beginning in 1958 and stretching into the 1970s, he traveled to Graz, Austria each summer to study thousands of autopsy reports (Graz is the capital of Styria, an Austrian province). By 1975, he had personally reviewed over 70,000 consecutive autopsy reports from the years 1930 through 1972.

In 1958, he met with Dr. Ratzenhofer, a pathologist, who was in charge of the ongoing autopsy studies in Graz. Dr. Barnes wasted little time in telling the doctor his theory that subnormal body temperatures were indicative of hypothyroidism, and that accelerated hardening of the arteries (atherosclerosis) was one of the principal manifestations of the illness. Before Dr. Barnes finished explaining his theories, the Austrian doctor interrupted, "Dr. Barnes, all of the people in Styria run low body temperatures and all suffer atherosclerosis."

From the first 10,000 autopsies studied, Dr. Barnes found only one person who was not suffering some degree of atherosclerosis. This included the very young who succumbed to infections or cancer. The autopsies revealed only one heart attack per 125 deaths occurred in 1930. By 1970, heart attacks had increased to one death in 14. This came about with little change in the Austrians' diet.

Drs. Barnes and Ratzenhofer were now ready to publish the true reason for the explosion of heart attacks in the twentieth century. They published their landmark study "The Role of Natural Consequences in the Changing Death Patterns" in *The Journal of the American Geriatrics Society* in 1974. The causes of death in 1930 were compared to those from 1970. The introduction of iodine supplementation (a trace element necessary for thyroid hormones), drugs to treat tuberculosis, and antibiotics occurred in the interim. However, a year-by-year study of the autopsies revealed very little change in death patterns until the introduction of antibiotics and antituberculin drugs after World War II. Therefore, most of these dramatic changes occurred in only 25 years (1945-1970).[20]

The comparisons from autopsy results in the publication are listed in Tables 3.1 and 3.2. Note the number of deaths are per 1,000 autopsies.

Table 3.1 **Phenomenal Rise in the Incidence of a Few Diseases According to Autopsies at Graz, Austria, Between 1930 and 1970 (number per 1,000 autopsies)**

Category	1930	1970	% Change
Heart attacks	6.8	69.0	+915
Emphysema	8.6	40.6	+372
Prostatic cancer	1.8	8.3	+361
Cancer in children	1.2	5.4	+349
Bronchial (lung) cancer	11.0	44.0	+300

Table 3.2 **Fluctuations in Various Categories of Deaths at Graz, Austria, 1930 and 1970 (number per 1,000 autopsies)**

Category	1930	1970	% Change
Deaths from infections	426	185	−56
Deaths from malignancies	189	240	+27
Deaths from degenerative diseases	238	343	+44
Deaths from accidents	37	47	+27

Source: Barnes, B., and Ratzenhofer, M. The Role of Natural Consequences in Changing Death Patterns, *Journal of the American Geriatrics Association* 1974; 22(6): 176-179. Reprinted with permission.

Over 42% of the deaths in 1930 resulted from infectious diseases. By 1970, deaths from infections had fallen to 18% of the total. Those patients who were susceptible to infections, i.e. the hypothyroid, were now surviving long enough to develop heart attacks, emphysema, malignancies, and other degenerative diseases associated with hypothyroidism. In 1930, only 47% of the total deaths were from patients over 50 years old. By 1970, total deaths for those over the age of 50 were 67%.

Heart disease and emphysema accounted for 90% of the increase in degenerative diseases. Emphysema has always been associated with recurrent infections. Its incidence increased 370%. Prostate cancer, juvenile cancer, and lung cancer accounted for 86% of the rise in malignant diseases. Historically, patients with tuberculosis (TB) were 20 times more likely to develop lung cancer than the general population. Eradicating TB allowed for a 300% increase in lung cancer.[20,21] The rate of rise in heart attacks paralleled the drop of deaths caused from infections. As long as infections took the lives of the young, heart attacks remained rare. Those escaping early death from other infections frequently succumbed to tuberculosis. Prior to the introduction of antituberculin drugs in 1944, the average age of deaths for tuberculosis victims was 38 years. My mother's grandfather died of TB at age 38. The average age for first heart attacks has remained in the 60s.

The etiology or cause of heart attacks was not described until 1912. Dr. Barnes' notes from medical school training, in the early 1930s, were almost devoid of disease from coronary (heart) arteries. It was a minor problem at that time. In 1870 deaths from tuberculosis in America had been 270 per 100,000. By 1900, the number of deaths was halved as a result of the introduction of sanatoria care (hospitals specifically caring for TB). However, this change resulted in a "new" population beginning to emerge who were susceptible to infections.[22]

The rate of heart attacks dropped precipitously in Europe during World War II. Graz was no exception. Most scientists and doctors attributed the decline to the wartime diet, one low in animal fat. The autopsies proved their theory wrong. The incidence of heart attacks in 1939, at the start of the war, was 12 per 1,000 autopsies. By 1945, there were only 3 deaths from heart attacks per 1,000. However, atherosclerosis in the aorta (our largest artery originating from the heart) and the blood vessels supplying the heart (coronary arteries) had doubled in severity among autopsied patients under the age of 50. The number of patients affected with atherosclerosis under 50 had also doubled. In other words, atherosclerosis had quadrupled in only six years. The elimination of animal fats and dairy products appeared to greatly accelerate atherosclerosis. If atherosclerosis was accelerated, then why the drop in heart attacks?

In 1939, there were 27 deaths from tuberculosis per 1,000 men between 30 and 60 years of age. In 1944, there were 55 deaths from TB per 1,000. Deaths from other infections also rose. The deaths from TB and other infections accounted for the drop from 12 to 3 deaths from heart attacks per 1,000 autopsies. Germany had a precipitous rise in TB during the war and a marked decline in heart attacks. Great Britain had a slight increase in TB and a slight decrease in heart attacks. TB and infections did not increase in America, thus heart attacks did not decline. Penicillin and drugs to treat TB were introduced in 1944, extending the life of patients. Heart attacks again spiraled upward.[22]

Can you guess what the autopsies from 1944 and 1945 revealed about the coronary arteries of those who died from TB? Severe atherosclerosis is correct. The Graz autopsies revealed advanced atherosclerosis in all of the patients who died from tuberculosis. Had they not died from tuberculosis, a heart attack likely would have ensued.

What do you think the 1947 autopsies revealed about those now dying from heart attacks? Their lungs were full of TB. The introduction of drugs to treat TB in 1944 allowed those suffering from the illness to survive long enough to succumb to a heart attack. It would seem diet had nothing to do with their deaths.

Dr. Barnes realized quite early in his career that hypothyroidism was pervasive and a majority of those afflicted were not being diagnosed or properly treated. By 1950, he also recognized his patients had not suffered any heart attacks while their incidence was exploding in the rest of America. In 1950, years before he discovered the existence of the Graz autopsies, Dr. Barnes began a long-term study to determine if proper treatment of hypothyroidism would prevent heart attacks.

Two years earlier, The National Heart Institute began the Framingham Study. It was officially named, "The Heart Disease Epidemiology Study." The objective: To determine why heart attacks were rapidly reaching epidemic proportions.

Over 5,000 adult residents of Framingham, Massachusetts volunteered to participate in the long-term medical study. The group underwent thorough physical exams. All were free of heart disease initially. Participants were examined at two year intervals. People who later suffered heart attacks helped determine the so-called "risk factors" that became associated with the illness. Risk factors included high blood pressure, elevated cholesterol, increasing age, and having a family history of heart attacks. Men were found to be at higher risk of heart attacks than women.

Dr. Barnes intended for his study to parallel the Framingham Study. Data from the ongoing Framingham Study was published every few years. In 1972, after 22 years of his ongoing study, Dr. Barnes published the results of his work in a book, *Heart Attack Rareness in Thyroid-Treated Patients*. The research included 1,569 patients who received treatment for their hypothyroidism. A minimum of two years of thyroid therapy was required to be included in the study. A number of these patients had been on thyroid medication for the entire study. An individual patient's symptoms, response to the hormones, and basal temperatures determined their dosage of thyroid hormones. The chart that follows shows the comparison between his patients and those from the Framingham Study.[4,22]

Table 3.3 **Comparison of the Framingham Study Prediction of Coronary Cases versus Dr. Barnes' Actual Cases Observed among His Patients**

Sex	Classification	# of Patients Treated	Patient Years	Study Coronary Prediction	Barnes' Actual Cases
F	Age 30-59	490	2,705	7.6	0
F	High risk*	172	1,086	7.3	0
F	Age over 60	182	955	7.8	0
M	Age 30-59	382	2,192	12.8	1
M	High risk*	186	1,070	18.5	2
M	Age over 60	157	816	18.0	1
	Totals	1,569	8,824	72.0	4

*High risk = high cholesterol, high blood pressure, or both.

Source: Barnes, B. *Hypothyroidism, the Unsuspected Illness*, Harper and Row, 1976. Page 180. Reprinted with permission.

Over 90% of predicted heart attacks from the Framingham Study were prevented.

The Framingham Study would have predicted that 72 of Dr. Barnes' patients should have suffered heart attacks. Only four occurred. In addition, at least 30 patients who quit the study and discontinued thyroid hormones suffered fatal heart attacks within six years of stopping their thyroid. Many of these patients had moved. Their new doctors declined to continue thyroid treatment. Blood tests often showed the patients did not need thyroid hormones. Others stopped taking their medication after their symptoms, such as acne, resolved.

Dr. Barnes purposely did not attempt to control cholesterol, smoking, exercise, or other variables among his study group. He wanted the only variable between his patients, and those from the Framingham Study, to be the use of thyroid hormones.

In 1976, four years after his book, *Heart Attack Rareness in Thyroid Treated Patients*, was published, Dr. Barnes published another ground breaking book, *Solved: The Riddle of Heart Attacks*. Despite the publication of eight editions through 1999, mainstream medicine continues to dismiss his irrefutable work.[23]

A study, published in *The New England Journal of Medicine* (August 24, 1998), found the incidence of first-time heart attacks among Americans appears to be on the rise. Dr. Barnes predicted that our massive effort to control heart attacks would fail, unless we recognized and properly treated hypothyroidism.

Supportive Research

Currently, around 900,000 Americans a year undergo angioplasty, where doctors insert a catheter to expand a blocked coronary artery. A tiny balloon is inflated at the obstruction in order to reopen the blocked artery. Following angioplasty, around 30% of these same coronary arteries clog up again within six months. If this occurs, another catheter is often used to place a stent (a spring-like, mesh device) in a further attempt to keep the clogged artery open. Stents reduce the reblockage rate from 25% to 15%.

Recent medical studies provide further support linking atherosclerosis to both infection and inflammation. In one study, 238 patients who required stents were randomly divided into two groups. One group received the standard stent. The other group received stents coated with an antibiotic. The coated stents slowly released the antibiotic for about 45 days. Twenty-six percent of the standard stent group suffered reblockage within six months. **None** of the group, whose stents were coated with antibiotics, suffered a recurrence.[24] This indicates that infection and inflammation have a causal effect on atherosclerosis.

In January 2002, researchers in Germany confirmed this by reporting that there is a significant association between the number of infections that a patient has suffered and the extent of atherosclerosis in the arteries in the heart, neck, and legs. Both bacterial and viral infections appeared to be involved. In this study, 572 patients with heart disease were followed for three years. Over the three year study, patients who tested positive for up to three types of infections had a death rate from heart disease of 3.1%. The death rate was 9.8% for those with four or five different infectious agents and 15% for those with six or eight.[25]

Do you think the doctors and scientists of the third millennium have all the answers when it comes to heart disease? I quote from a 1997 article from *The New England Journal of Medicine* entitled, "Shattuck Lecture – Cardiovascular Medicine at the Turn of the Millennium: Triumphs, Concerns, and Opportunities." From the article's section entitled, "Inadequate Knowledge," "Although much has been learned about the causes of coronary heart disease, the gaps in knowledge are noteworthy; for example, **fully half of all patients with this condition do not have any of the established coronary risk factors**."[26] The primary risk factors include hypertension, elevated cholesterol, cigarette smoking, diabetes mellitus, marked obesity, and physical inactivity.

At the 2001 American Public Health Association meeting, I asked a prominent cardiologist if this fact bothered her. Her response, "Well, it's hard to measure stress." Apparently, she felt assured that "stress" was the causative factor in the other 50% of heart attacks. Stress is an important factor in the development of generalized immune suppression and increased incidence of disease. In those who suffer hypothyroidism, additional thyroid hormones fortify the immune system and greatly aid our body's ability to withstand stress. If stress were the underlying causative factor in heart attacks, then they would have been a major problem prior to the twentieth century.

A study published in February, 2002 in *The New England Journal of Medicine* involving almost 28,000 patients and covering eight years, revealed that elevated low density "bad" cholesterol levels were not as important in predicting heart attacks as C-reactive protein (CRP). CRP is an indicator of the amount of inflammation in our bodies including the blood vessels. Elevated CRP was also related to the development of diabetes. Again, more hard evidence has been provided to support Dr. Barnes' work.

The lead story in the February 23, 2004 issue of *Time* magazine was devoted to inflammation. An explosion of research has linked heart attacks, cancer, Alzheimer's, and a multitude of other diseases to the presence of inflammation in the body. Huge amounts of money and research flow into the study of anti-inflammatory drugs such as aspirin and their effects on our most common diseases.

New to this research are the statin drugs currently used to treat elevated cholesterol. They have been proven to decrease inflammation as well as cholesterol. The diminished inflammation may be the main reason these drugs decrease the risk of heart attacks. In addition, the side effect profiles from these statin drugs are not good. Well over 100 people died from one of the new statins, which was quickly pulled off the market.

The desired statins' effect, to lower cholesterol and decrease inflammation, was seen in patients taking desiccated thyroid. I believe the decrease in cholesterol contributes little to statins' effectiveness. My patients, who have maintained desiccated thyroid for at least one year, have consistently low levels of inflammation as measured by their CRP. Normal thyroid metabolism prevents recurrent infections and inhibits chronic inflammation.

> For more information: Dr. Barnes chronicled the history and relation between hypothyroidism, infections, atherosclerosis, and heart attacks in his books, *Heart Attack Rareness in Thyroid-Treated Patients* and *Solved: The Riddle of Heart Attacks*. These two books and their bibliographies are the Rosetta Stone for comprehending the cause and prevention of heart attacks.[22,23]

The Value of Case Studies

Doctors, as well as lay people who read Dr. Barnes' book, *Hypothyroidism, the Unsuspected Illness*, often complain his research is only a compilation of individual patient case studies. Beginning in the twentieth century, doctors and scientists began to insist upon "double-blind studies" to prove the efficacy of drugs. Let me explain the meaning of a double-blind study. Doctors compare one drug with another drug. Some studies compare a drug with an inert (inactive) substance called a placebo. The drugs and/or placebo both have an identical appearance to ensure that neither the doctor nor patient can discern any difference. Only the people in charge of the investigation know who gets the drug or the placebo. The reason is to avoid any bias the doctor might impart if he or she knew what the patient received. These studies may last from several months to several years.

The number of people required for these studies varies. For instance, if one drug is known to be effective in 50% of patients, and the other drug is thought to be effective in 75% of patients, the number of patients necessary to be statistically significant would have to be relatively large. If a new drug were compared to a placebo, the study may not require as much time or as many patients. However, placebos may affect up to 30% of patients as a result of just being involved in the study process (the power of the mind is a long way from being understood). This is known as the "placebo effect".

Until recent data to the contrary emerged, double-blind studies were thought to be far superior to case studies. In a case study, patients are given a known drug and their progress or outcome is reported. The results of case studies have been thought to be clouded by the patient and doctor biases as well as the placebo effect.

In January, 2000, a research paper was published in *The New England Journal of Medicine* entitled, "A Comparison of Observational Studies and Randomized, Controlled Trials." The study concluded, "The results of well-designed observational studies do not systematically overestimate the magnitude of the effects of treatment as compared with those in randomized, controlled trials on the same topic." The randomized, controlled trial is a double-blind study. Observational studies are the same as case studies. In other words, a well-designed case study is just as valid as a double-blind study.[27]

This indicates that Dr. Barnes' long-term studies, covering decades and involving thousands of patients, are sound. Any doubts about the validity of Dr. Barnes' comparison of his group of patients with the Framingham Study group are simply not realistic.

In 1973, Dr. Barnes published another landmark paper in *The Journal of the American Geriatric Society* entitled, "On the Genesis of Atherosclerosis." He outlined most of the aforementioned remarks as well as many literature citations by other researchers supporting his observations in this publication.[28] Interestingly, the very next article following his landmark study in this journal was, "A Surgeon Reviews a Half-Century of Progress in the Treatment of Coronary Artery Disease." All of the dogma concerning heart disease, which persists in today's medical literature, was captured in that article. Heredity, diet, cholesterol, smoking, diabetes, and high blood pressure were all to blame. Autopsies showing the presence of atherosclerosis in young American military men killed in Korea and other regions were noted. Whereas, it noted that there was a lack of atherosclerosis in Chinese, Japanese, and Korean soldiers killed.[29] Dr. Mazel, the author, assumed the reason for the lack of atherosclerosis in the Asian countries was due to heredity and the lack of saturated fats in their diet. He was not aware the rate of tuberculosis in these countries was comparable at the time to America's level during the nineteenth century.

Drs. Barnes' and Ratzenhofer's paper, "The Role of Natural Consequences in the Changing Death Patterns," included a listing from the World Health Organization on the distribution of the sexes in deaths from tuberculosis for the years 1947 to 1949 in several countries.

Table 3.4   **TB Deaths per 100,000**

Country	Males	Females
Japan	169	129
Italy	59	38
England	53	33
Canada	34	28
U.S. (whites)	30	14

Source: Barnes, B. O., Ratzenhofer, M., and Gisi, R. The Role of Natural Consequences in the Changing Death Patterns. *Journal American of the American Geriatrics Society* 1974; 22: 176. Reprinted with permission.

This shows us that the Asian hypothyroid population was dying from tuberculosis and other infections just like those from Graz in 1930. Thanks to TB, they did not live long enough to develop lethal coronary artery disease as compared to the Americans. Therefore, the lower incidence of heart attacks almost certainly did not result from their diet.

Dr. Barnes made special note in his research and lecture tapes regarding the lack of heart attacks in underprivileged third world countries. Without exception, deaths from infectious disease accounted for the scarcity of heart attacks. The bibliographies from his books list many such studies that included autopsy findings.

Drs. Barnes and Ratzenhofer concluded their research paper by stating: "It is fitting that the tuberculosis sanatoriums of the past are being converted into general hospitals for the management of heart attacks. The identical patients are being cared for, but they are arriving 25 years later with a new ailment."[20]

Chapter 4
Diabetes

Dr. Barnes believed diabetes was due in large part to hypo-thyroidism. New cases of diabetes were extremely rare among his large group of patients being treated for hypothyroidism. He thought the recurrent infections and impaired immune, hormonal, and internal organ functions the hypothyroid suffered from resulted in diabetes as well as a myriad other chronic illnesses. He also predicted the incidence of diabetes would balloon, along with the increased incidence and severity of hypothyroidism.

The rate of diabetes in America increased almost 50% from 1990 to 1998. Researchers blamed the increased incidence on genetic predisposition, increasing obesity, and declining physical activity. However, a report from the Centers for Disease Control (March 2001) revealed the level of physical activity in America did not change between 1990 and 1998. The report also stated racial differences were minimal, regarding exercise habits, yet minorities suffer a higher incidence of diabetes.

There are two predominant forms of diabetes. The most severe is Type 1, which has a peak at 12 years of age. It occurs when the pancreas abruptly stops secreting insulin, blood sugar levels skyrocket, and exogenous (prescription) insulin is necessary to maintain life. Diabetes researchers have blamed viruses, autoimmune factors, and genetic factors for this type of diabetes.

Type 2 diabetes is characterized by a gradual onset, which usually begins between 50 and 60 years of age. Cellular receptors become resistant to insulin despite often-adequate secretion of insulin by the pancreas. This is the type of diabetes that has been attributed to lack of exercise, genetic predisposition, and obesity. Type 2 diabetes accounts for over 90% of the total diabetics.

In 1970, according to Dr. Barnes, around 2% of the U.S. population suffered diabetes (Types 1 and 2). In Graz, Austria, where hypothyroidism was endemic, the rate was 4% at that time. The number of diabetics in our country has now ballooned to around 16 million, which is over 5%. The American Diabetic Association estimates another five million are diabetic who have not yet been diagnosed. Type 2 diabetes was formerly termed "adult onset diabetes". However, the illness is suddenly appearing among our young, and its incidence is rapidly rising.

Most people do not realize that almost all the complications that result from diabetes are due to hardening of the arteries or atherosclerosis. These complications include blindness, kidney failure, heart attacks, gangrene, and nerve damage. Diabetics suffer accelerated atherosclerosis identical to that associated with hypothyroidism.

In 1970, autopsy studies showed the rate of amputations in the non-diabetic population in Graz, Austria was five times that of the diabetic population in the United States. Antibiotics and antituberculin drugs allowed Austria's endemic hypothyroid population to survive. Hence, their overall rate of atherosclerosis was much worse than America's.

While new cases of diabetes were very rare among Dr. Barnes' patients who were being treated for hypothyroidism, a significant number of patients with diabetes sought his help. After many years of practice, he finally realized that **none of his patients with diabetes had developed any of the typical and more advanced complications from their illness.** Dr. Barnes researched old medical literature in an attempt to find out if there were any other reports to support these findings. There was a study that had been ignored since 1954. It was entitled "Coexistence of Hypothyroidism with Diabetes Mellitus" by Crosby D. Eaton M.D. The study included several hundred diabetic patients of all ages who were treated for years. Dr. Eaton realized the vast majority of his diabetic patients also suffered hypothyroidism. He administered desiccated thyroid hormones with no adverse affect upon their diabetic control. He reported a vastly reduced incidence of complications related to diabetes as well as the elimination of the symptoms associated with hypothyroidism.[30]

Dr. Barnes was not the first to report what now seems to be an astonishing revelation. However, he was the first doctor to back up his report with hard evidence consisting of 70,000 autopsy studies and long-term patient outcome studies. Yet, the medical community continues to minimize the importance of these reports. The status quo for the control of diabetes and its complications continues to be the manipulation of blood sugar levels. Once the complications from accelerated atherosclerosis begin, numerous and heroic attempts by the medical community directed at symptomatic treatment are usually implemented.

Dr. Barnes presented his research on the coexistence of diabetes and hypothyroidism at a 1971 American Medical Association meeting. He also met with prominent doctors at our nation's most prestigious institutions. Unfortunately, he found no sympathetic ears, despite the wealth of evidence he had gathered from the autopsies, his own patients, and Dr. Eaton's report. He pleaded for further studies, but none would be forthcoming. Dr. Barnes' lectures and books address the subject. His lecture tapes are available through his research foundation.[10]

The effort and money wasted since Dr. Eaton's and Dr. Barnes' publications, as well as the toll of human suffering, is extremely disconcerting. Over 50 years have passed since Dr. Eaton's report and 35 years since Dr. Barnes'. With the passage of time and distinguished careers, medical dogma becomes more entrenched while mainstream medicine remains unchanged.

In my opinion, every diabetic patient seen in my practice has suffered hypothyroidism. The family histories usually reveal the profound hereditary influence of hypothyroidism.

In summary, our new, susceptible to infection population has escaped early death thanks to the great marvels of modern medicine. Just one hundred years ago, half the population in all of "Western Civilization" died from infection at an early age. Two hundred years ago, the figures were much higher. Scientists and doctors have dismissed the influence of genetics as the cause for our explosion of chronic illnesses. They cannot fathom how our genes and the inner workings of our cells could change so dramatically in such a brief period of time. In fact, by preserving weakened immune systems, which were previously flushed out of the gene pool through the millennia, this is indeed the case. The following chapter will offer further evidence and recent research findings. This new, longer surviving hypothyroid population goes on to develop atherosclerosis as well as the broad range of other degenerative diseases associated with hypothyroidism. Without prompt intervention, our offspring are doomed to suffer even more problems. The explosion of childhood illnesses, including skyrocketing mental aberrations and diabetes, is a gloomy testimonial to the accuracy of Dr. Barnes' predictions.

The Broda O. Barnes M.D. Research Foundation can provide a referral list of physicians who embrace the tenets put forth by Dr. Barnes at:

www.brodabarnes.org

203 261-2101 USA

Chapter 5
Hypothyroidism: Type 1 versus Type 2

In order to clarify my understanding of thyroid diseases to you, Dr. Boc and I have defined Type 1 hypothyroidism as failure of the thyroid gland to produce sufficient amounts of thyroid hormones necessary to maintain "normal" blood levels of those hormones and "normal" blood levels of the thyroid stimulating hormone (TSH) produced by the pituitary gland. The TSH is the standard blood test your doctor checks when looking for hypothyroidism (see Chapter 7 for a detailed discussion of thyroid lab tests). Around five percent of Americans suffer Type 1 hypothyroidism.

Dr. Boc and I defined Type 2 hypothyroidism as peripheral resistance to thyroid hormones at the cellular level. It is not due to a lack of thyroid hormones. Normal amounts of thyroid hormones and thyroid stimulating hormone (TSH) are usually detected by blood tests; therefore, **blood tests do not detect Type 2 hypothyroidism.** Type 2 hypothyroidism is usually inherited. However, environmental toxins may also cause or exacerbate the problem. The pervasiveness of Type 2 hypothyroidism has yet to be recognized by mainstream medicine but already is in epidemic proportions.

Western Civilization recognized hypothyroidism as one of the most widespread and severe medical problems in the late nineteenth and early twentieth centuries. Several of the world's great medical centers, such as those in Vienna and Berlin, were located in severely affected areas. Consequently, hypothyroidism was one of the most thoroughly investigated diseases.

Two conditions associated with hypothyroidism, goiter and cretinism, must be clarified to illustrate this point. A goiter is an abnormal enlargement of the thyroid gland causing swelling in the neck where the thyroid gland is located. The word "goiter" is derived from the Latin "gutter," meaning throat. Production of thyroid hormones requires iodine, which makes iodine an essential element in our diet. Without sufficient iodine, the thyroid gland may enlarge in an often vain attempt to produce the normal amount of thyroid hormones. Historically, goiters commonly occurred where iodine content in the soil and drinking water was low. Mountainous regions and lands scoured by glaciers were particularly affected prior to the introduction of iodized salt. The result was chronic hypothyroidism and goiters in regions low in iodine. Goiters may grow strikingly large. They can compress the trachea (breathing), esophagus (swallowing), and blood vessels and nerves to the head. You can imagine the resultant complications. Babies born without thyroid function fail to develop mentally, sexually, and remain severely retarded dwarfs. These unfortunate people are called cretins. The following picture is taken from the first medical textbook devoted to diseases of the endocrine glands. The patient is a cretin with a large goiter.

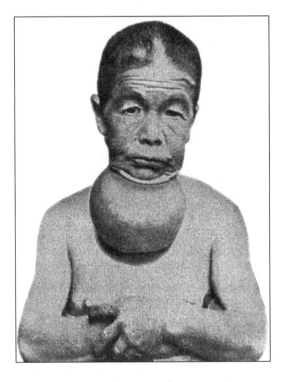

Source: Zondek, H. 1944. *Diseases of the Endocrine Glands*, 4th ed. Baltimore: The Williams and Wilkins Company. Reprinted with permission.

The derivation of "cretin" is Swiss-French from the Latin "Christus" (Christ). "Christian mentally challenged" is the Encarta Dictionary's definition. As early as 1800, doctors began to express the view that goiter was the first level and cretinism the last and worst degree of the same degenerative condition. That condition was found to be hypothyroidism in the late nineteenth century.

Hermann Zondek M.D., was a giant in the early study of hypothyroidism and endocrine disease. His accomplishments included the first successful treatment of heart failure with thyroid hormones in 1918. In the early 1920s, he published one of the first textbooks about diseases of the endocrine glands and their treatment.[8,31] A paragraph from Dr. Zondek's famous textbook (translated from German into English in 1944), *Diseases of the Endocrine Glands*, illustrated the pervasiveness of hypothyroidism in the early twentieth century.

"In several of the countries mentioned goitre is one of the severest national scourges. In some of the worst affected districts of <u>Styria</u> [Austria] there are over 1,000 cretins per 100,000 inhabitants. An important form of the disease is the juvenile type, beginning mostly in puberty, between the 14th and 16th year. According to reliable statistics, 40% to 50% of the schoolchildren in Tyrol and southern Bavaria are affected; in some parts of Switzerland the figure is 90%. For Bern, Wegelin [a Swiss doctor] estimates the incidence of congenital goitre at 66%. In Vienna well-marked goitre was found in one of nine, manifest thyroid enlargement in 44% of the schoolchildren. Among 11,000 New York schoolgirls of varying ages, 20.3% had enlarged thyroids. In goitre regions children are evidently exposed to a far greater risk of acquiring the disease than adults. The tendency to goitre seems to be inherited."[8]

The Styria to which Dr. Zondek referred is the province in Austria whose capital is Graz. Graz is where Dr. Barnes studied over 70,000 autopsy results (refer to Chapter 3).

There were iodine deficient regions and abundant goiters in America as well. The introduction of iodized salt in 1918 resulted in the sudden need for many people to have goiter removal surgery. A small percentage of people with goiters became <u>hyper</u>thyroid when given iodine. When provided with iodine, their enlarged thyroid glands produced too many hormones. <u>Hyper</u>thyroidism results in rapid heart rates, weight loss, sweating, diarrhea, insomnia, elevated temperatures, and death if untreated. The Mayo Clinic, Leahey Clinic, and several other major medical centers were constructed because of the large amount of delicate thyroid surgery required to alleviate the resultant epidemic of <u>hyper</u>thyroidism in America. As a result of the American experience, Europeans were slower to introduce iodine because of the feared consequences. Austria delayed widespread introduction until the 1960s.

Eugene Hertoghe M.D., was a member of The Royal Academy of Medicine of Belgium and the first doctor to describe the "abortive" (mild) forms of hypothyroidism. Three successive generations of Hertoghe endocrinologists have followed in his footsteps. Therese Hertoghe M.D., his great-granddaughter, is currently among the most renowned experts on hypothyroidism in the world.

The senior Dr. Hertoghe addressed the 1914 International Surgical Congress in New York (copies of this lecture are available through the Barnes Foundation). I quote from the lecture:

> The weakness of the thyroid gland is usually hereditary, and it is rare that one does not find traces of milder defect among the ascending, descending, or collateral relations of a person suffering from well-marked myxedema. One must inquire carefully into the family history; it will be found an inexhaustible source of information regarding symptoms which will render one more familiar with the milder cases of hypothyroidism.[32]

Dr. Hertoghe recognized the illness occurred spontaneously or may be inherited. He stated, "From all this we may conclude that thyroid weakness is very frequent, at least in a mild form."[32]

He went on to say, "Infiltration is the constant lesion of thyroid deficiency [referring to myxedema or thickening of the skin and connective tissue]. A most constant symptom of myxedema is a lowering of the temperature. The patient is in a state of habitual chilliness, showing itself in women and children by constant coldness of the hands and feet." Hypothyroid adult males are not as prone to feeling cold, which may be due to their much higher levels of testosterone.

Natural Selection Defeated

The number of people affected by hypothyroidism has been greatly magnified by the tremendous strides in medicine made during the twentieth century. Since the dawn of mankind, much of the population never survived childbirth, dying during infancy, childhood, or adolescence.

Early death and susceptibility to infection are hallmarks of hypothyroidism. Infants and the young, who were susceptible to infectious diseases, died, failing to pass on their weak genes. Throughout the millennia, survival of the fittest kept the hypothyroid gene pool under control.

Austrian medicine had come a long way since the eighteenth century. In Graz, 98 out of every 100 consecutive newborns had failed to survive when Empress Maria Theresa mandated autopsies. Prenatal deaths remained high through the last years when Dr. Barnes reviewed autopsies. In 1972, prenatal deaths in infants accounted for 8.5% of the total deaths for the year (these were not included in the other deaths due to infections that same year). Miscarriages and prenatal deaths are also indicative of hypothyroidism, which help control its pervasiveness.

Dr. Barnes studied the Hunza, an ancient civilization of people who inhabit the mountains of Kashmir. Chronic illnesses such as arthritis, heart disease, atherosclerosis, diabetes, cancer, stomach problems, high blood pressure, and obesity were conspicuously absent among the Hunza. They lived vigorous lives well past the age of 100. It had been their custom over the centuries for the mother to nurse male babies until the age of three and female children until the age of two. If the children were unable to nurse and thrive, they died. Dr. Barnes attributed the Hunza's excellent health and longevity to an unusually healthy endocrine system. Those with hypothyroidism and weak immune systems died in their infancy.

A British doctor named McCarrison, stationed near Kashmir in the early twentieth century, noted the absence of goiters in the Hunza population while many of the surrounding peoples suffered a high frequency. Dr. Barnes studied McCarrison's writings and cited one instance when tuberculosis was introduced into the Hunza's isolated society. TB is an airborne disease that spreads quickly in susceptible populations. However, in the Hunza, a few mild cases resulted without any deaths. This was in stark contrast to other civilizations such as the American Indians, Eskimos, and countless others who were devastated by the introduction of TB.

Eliminating early death from infection has greatly changed our gene pool and destinies. A brief review of the recorded history of infectious diseases' toll may help to illustrate the magnitude of this change.

Since the dawn of recorded history, smallpox epidemics brought down entire civilizations. The first known epidemic was recorded after the Egyptian-Hittite war in 1350 B.C. (the Hittites and Egyptians were the two superpowers of their time). Egyptian mummies, prior to the war, showed that the disease had not shown deference (favor) to the mighty Pharaohs.

After the Hittites were exposed to smallpox, their population was so impacted that Egypt reigned supreme thereafter. However, the Egyptians' average life span was only 35 years. Yet, their ancient mummies show evidence of arthritis, atherosclerosis, and telltale signs of smallpox or other infections. This tells us that hypothyroidism has been pervasive for thousands of years. The relationship between arthritis and hypothyroidism will be discussed in Chapters 8 and 10.

The population of Mexico is estimated to have fallen from about 25 million to 1.6 million after the Spanish introduced smallpox to the New World. America's native population suffered equally. Many American slaves came from areas in Africa where smallpox and goiters were endemic. Smallpox also had a predilection for children. At least 300 million people worldwide lost their lives during the twentieth century before it was eradicated. Our hypothyroid population would be decimated should it return.

The Bubonic Plague was known as the "Black Death" during Renaissance Europe. After it appeared in 1338, one-third to one-half of the population of Europe died in just two years. Recurrent plague continued to claim the lives of a large percentage of children for the next 300 years.

The Great Flu Pandemic of 1918-1919 killed almost 10% of the American population. Again, the victims of preference were the young and old with weak immune systems. One of my family's neighbors lost four of her six children.

Tuberculosis remained the "Captain of Death" well into the twentieth century. In 1870, deaths from TB were 270 per 100,000 of the U.S. population. Western Europe had higher rates, due to increased crowding in their more numerous and larger cities. By 1900, due to the introduction of sanatorium care for TB victims, the death rate was halved. However, TB remained the leading cause of death in America, among the 16 to 39 year-old age group, well into the 1930s.

How many of us have survived to reproduce because of the introduction of antibiotics in 1944? Interestingly, the first mass production of penicillin was used for the troops who participated in the Allied Invasion of Normandy during World War II. Bacteriologist and British Nobel Laureate, Sir Alexander Fleming, first discovered penicillin in 1928. Dr. Fleming was unable to convince skeptical colleagues of the importance of his discovery. He could not produce sufficient quantities of penicillin necessary to eradicate severe infections. He did attain temporary remissions in a number of patients dying from infections. Frustrated, he saved a sample of the penicillium mold from which the drug derived. British doctors feverishly searched the medical literature during World War II in their quest to find an antibiotic. They happened upon Dr. Fleming's report. The bottle of penicillium mold had remained on his shelf for over a decade. The British doctors used his mold to begin the production of penicillin for the second time.

Have you deduced the origin of hypothyroidism yet? It appears to have been a tremendous problem since the dawn of civilization. It may be part of nature's "survival of the fittest" scheme.

Gone are the plagues, as well as smallpox and tuberculosis, which are now controlled by improved sanitation and vaccinations. The introduction of penicillin, followed by generations of antibiotics, antifungal, and antiviral drugs were the final straw. Consequently, there has been a tremendous reduction of deaths from infection among our young. Prior to the dawn of antibiotics and the near elimination of death from infections in our young, children with more severe forms of Type 2 hypothyroidism and weakened immune systems rarely survived into adulthood.

Those who escape death from infection are the "new population" who suffer Type 2 hypothyroidism. Their numbers mushroomed during the twentieth century. This population continues to pass on their predilection to infection and hypothyroidism to increasingly larger numbers.

The Incidence of Hypothyroidism

Dr. Barnes cited Dr. Paul Starr from the University of Southern California as one of America's prominent early pioneers in the study of hypothyroidism. Dr. Starr estimated its incidence to be about 10% in the 1920s. However, I believe its incidence may have been much higher. Those affected with the illness were dying from infectious diseases. In 1915, Dr. Hertoghe stated, "The slighter forms of thyroid inadequacy are almost invariably missed; yet, owing to their extreme prevalence, the recognition of these is particularly important."[2]

Dr. Barnes organized a student health service at the University of Denver in 1941. He began the "Basal Temperature versus Basal Metabolism Study," which was later published in *The Journal of the American Medical Association*. Dr. Barnes found evidence of hypothyroidism in about 20% of the students.[9]

In 1976, after 35 more years of medical practice, research, and treating the increasingly aging population, he estimated its incidence in America to be 40%. He predicted the number would reach 50% by 1986. How could he arrive at these figures?

Dr. Barnes' 70,000 autopsy studies had proven the incidence of hypothyroidism and its associated stigmata increased in direct proportion to the decrease in deaths from infectious disease. At the turn of the nineteenth century, 50% of Americans were dying from infections at an early age. On Dr. Barnes' lecture tapes, he stated that 99 times out of 100, children who suffer frequent infections are hypothyroid. My patients continue to confirm his observations.

When an inherited disease reaches 50% of the population, it does not require a mathematician to calculate how fast the incidence will rise. In 1989, while lecturing at the Barnes Foundation annual meeting, Dr. Jacques Hertoghe, the third generation endocrinologist, estimated the incidence to be 80% among his Belgian countrymen. My observations and research support the conclusions of Drs. Barnes and Hertoghe.

Type 2 hypothyroidism is usually inherited and is insidious. There are no blood tests available to detect its presence. The diagnosis is made from the family's medical history, the patient's medical history, the physical exam, and the basal temperature. Type 1 hypothyroidism, the failure of the thyroid gland to produce "normal" amounts of thyroid hormones, affects around 5% of Americans and can be detected by blood tests. However, Type 1 hypothyroidism often develops in patients with underlying Type 2 hypothyroidism. You will read about how Type 2 hypothyroidism has a deleterious effect on hormone-producing glands and tissues in the next chapter. The familial predilection to develop Type 1 hypothyroidism is well established. The familial predilection to inherit hypothyroidism (Type 2) was described a century ago. Unfortunately, its prevalence has yet to be recognized by modern medicine.

Case Study

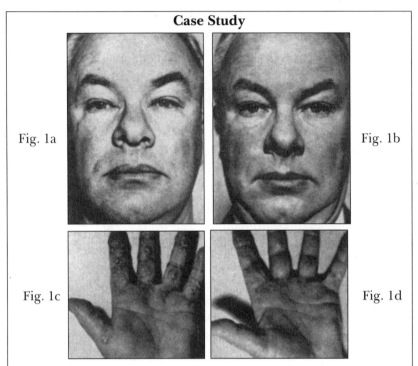

Fig. 1a

Fig. 1b

Fig. 1c

Fig. 1d

Source: Lisser, H., and Escamilla, R. F. Atlas of Clinical Endocrinology: Including Text of Diagnosis and Treatment. C.V. Mosby Company, 1957. Reprinted with permission.

Figure 1a. Myxedema in 49 year-old man, with widespread xanthomatous [cholesterol] lesions, developed over period of 18 months. Admitted fatigue, constipation, and cold intolerance. Had brassy voice, macroglossia [enlarged tongue], slow speech, bilateral nerve deafness; liver enlarged to 6 cm (23/8 in.) below right costal margin. BMR -35%; cholesterol, 926 mg %. Note puffiness of all features and narrow eye slits.

Figure 1b. Appearance of same patient after 3 months treatment with thyroid 1 1/2 grains (0.1 gm) daily. Note widened palpebral apertures [eyes], more alert expression, and sharpened features. BMR +8%; cholesterol, 196 mg %.

Figure 1c and d. Note characteristic xanthomatous nodules on hand which disappeared after thyroid therapy.

Chapter 6
The Energy Factories Within Our Cells:
Type 2 Hypothyroidism

Each and every cell in our bodies contains hundreds of mitochondria. What are mitochondria, and why are they so important?

Mitochondria are the principal sites where our bodies produce energy. These are literally microscopic energy factories that convert the food we eat into the chemical currency that our bodies use to function. If the body runs out of food, mitochondria may conveniently convert our own muscle protein or fat into energy. Mitochondria are responsible for about 90% of the energy production that cells and therefore, our tissues, organs, and bodies require for metabolism.

Do you think there may be a link between thyroid hormones and mitochondria? Recall from the first chapter that thyroid hormones are responsible for our metabolism. When thyroid hormones are given to animals, trillions of mitochondria increase in size and number. The total membrane surface of the mitochondria increases almost directly in proportion to the increased metabolic rate of the whole animal. My medical school textbook, *The Textbook of Medical Physiology*, **states, "It seems almost to be an obvious deduction that the principal function of thyroxine [thyroid hormone] might be simply to increase the number and activity of mitochondria."**[33]

Mitochondrial DNA are inherited solely from the mother. The mother's egg contains the entire set of DNA responsible for their production. This DNA is completely separate from the 46 chromosomes that define a person's individuality. Men's sperm contributes nothing in the replication or production of mitochondria. As stated in the initial report from 1888, hypothyroidism is chiefly inherited from the mother as well. In my experience, this holds particularly true for Type 2 hypothyroidism.

Whole biochemistry departments and teams of scientists are now devoted to the study of mitochondria. Several medical and scientific journals are also devoted to the same. Doctors and scientists rightfully import great significance to the function, or more aptly, the dysfunction of our mitochondria. However, these scientists all continue to overlook the correlation with hypothyroidism.

The American Academy of Anti-Aging meeting was held in Las Vegas, Nevada, December, 2000. Suzanne De La Monte M.D., recipient of the 2000 Alzheimer Research Medal, was an expert speaker on Alzheimer's disease.

Dr. De La Monte's lecture addressed the current understanding of Alzheimer's disease:

1. Energy metabolism is decreased in the mitochondria.
2. The amount of enzyme formation in these patients' mitochondria is also decreased.
3. The number of mitochondria is decreased.
4. Females are affected more than males.
5. The incidence is much higher in developed nations with lower early death rates.
6. The incidence increases with age.

Amazingly, all six of these problems associated with mitochondria are consistent with hypothyroidism. Several drugs and chemicals were mentioned to help rescue the aging brain. However, thyroid hormones were not among them.

I could not wait to speak to the doctor after her lecture. She and a doctor standing with her unknowingly answered the question that I had only dreamed of solving. Not only is the mitochondria DNA inherited solely from the mother, but this DNA suffers progressive damage throughout women's lives. The damage results in further mutations in the mitochondrial DNA. These mutations are cumulative and therefore, increase in number with each successive generation. In other words, each new generation escaping the rigors of survival of the fittest will suffer more health problems than the last.

Half of Americans over 85 suffer Alzheimer's. The vast majority of the patients in Dr. Barnes' study group lived into their 80s and 90s with all of their faculties remaining intact. Hypothyroidism impairs mitochondria, circulation, and limits the supply of vital nutrients to all the nerves including those in the brain. Any bets on the basal temperatures and history of other hypothyroid symptomatology in Alzheimer's patients and their families?

Several generations have now escaped early death from infections. The weak and defective mitochondrial DNA continues to be propagated. These energy factories upon which our basic metabolism depend become more weakened each successive generation. The principal way to help these mitochondria regain their function is to stimulate their activity and numbers by taking thyroid hormones.

Dr. De La Monte and her colleague were kind enough to give me a reference in the *Scientific American* (August, 1997) on page 40, "Mitochondrial DNA in Aging and Disease" by Douglas C. Wallace Ph.D. While reading the article, I realized this was the reason why hypothyroidism is inherited chiefly from the mother. This also explains why the severity of the illness continues to worsen. The article begins with a case history of a child affected by defective mitochondria:

At age five a seemingly healthy boy inexplicably began to lose his hearing, which disappeared entirely before he turned 18. In the interim, he was diagnosed as hyperactive and suffered occasional seizures. By the time he was 23, his vision had declined; he had cataracts, glaucoma, and progressive deterioration of the retina. Within five years he had experienced severe seizures, and his kidneys had failed. He died at 28 from his kidney disorder and a systemic infection.[34]

Mutations in the mitochondrial DNA are associated with heart failure, diabetes, the aging process, chronic degenerative illnesses such as Alzheimer's disease, and various motor (neurological or muscular) disturbances. **"Eventually, it became clear that the tissues and organs most readily affected by cellular energy declines [in order of impact] are the central nervous system, followed, in descending order of sensitivity, by heart and skeletal muscle, the kidneys, and 'hormone-producing' tissues."**[34] Once again, these are the same organs and tissues most often affected by hypothyroidism. Dr. Sonkin termed hypothyroidism not detected by blood tests as "symptomatic low metabolism".[6]

In 1995, The National Institutes of Health published a study involving 104 patients with a genetically inherited form of hypothyroidism that involved resistance to thyroid hormone in the thyroid hormone receptor gene. The tissue resistance involved, in descending order, the pituitary gland (one of our most important endocrine glands), the brain (the mainstay of our central nervous system), the bone, the liver, and the heart. In other words, the central nervous system, the heart, and an endocrine tissue were the most affected organs. **The symptoms the patients suffered with Type 2 hypothyroidism were the same as those with defects in their mitochondria.**[35]

In Dr. Zondek's landmark text, *The Diseases of the Endocrine Glands*, he described disturbances in growth (primarily bone abnormalities resulting from inadequate thyroid stimulus), anomalies in genital development (controlled by endocrine glands), and signs of mental disturbance (the central nervous system) as "the factors chiefly governed by the thyroid gland".[8]

In one of his publications, Dr. Sonkin cited a book, *Thyroid Disease and Muscle Dysfunction*, by Ian Ramsay M.D. Dr. Ramsay cited a number of studies concerning the alterations in human muscle tissues, which occur as result of hypothyroidism. In his chapter, "Muscle Abnormalities of Hypothyroidism," he discusses the unusual deformities found in mitochondria that are within the muscles.[36]

Dr. Wallace's *Scientific American* article about mitochondria continues, "Investigators have uncovered several remarkable features of the syndromes that spring from defects in the mitochondrial DNA. For instance, these conditions are often inherited, though not in the same way as disorders issuing from mutations in nuclear genes. And the resulting symptoms are more unpredictable than those caused by nuclear genetic mutations." Nuclear genes are determined by the chromosomes (genetic material) donated from both parents. Dr. Wallace also stated, "People born with mitochondrial DNA mutations often become ill only after a delay of years or sometimes decades, and their conditions usually worsen over time."[34]

In my opinion, this landmark article on mitochondrial mutations unwittingly and clearly described Type 2 hypothyroidism, i.e. the "Peripheral Resistance Syndrome" that Drs. Sonkin and Barnes believed responsible for the vast majority of hypothyroidism. The inheritance pattern described by The Clinical Society of London's report on myxedema in 1888 stated, "It is certain that in some cases there is direct transmission from the father or the mother, **chiefly from the latter**."[1] The mother's medical history is remarkably more consistent with hypothyroidism in the vast majority of the Type 2 hypothyroid patients I interviewed.

Mitochondrial mutations appear to be largely responsible for the metabolic defects at the cellular level, which result in a hypothyroid-like condition. Modern thyroid blood tests do not detect this because thyroid hormone levels may be normal, but they are not high enough to stimulate the genetically defective mitochondria into normal activity. The increased basal temperature that results from administering desiccated thyroid is a direct result of enhanced mitochondrial activity.

Another example of the profound influence that mitochondria may exert was aired in a special series about evolution on public television in 2001. One segment dealt with the growing problem of infertility in America. One in six American couples suffer fertility problems. In vitro fertilization aids a small number of people with infertility. Despite all of the hugely expensive and painful treatments, a large percentage of couples are unable to produce a child.

I was amazed to see the newest technique to aid these struggling couples' embryos' survival was to borrow a healthy donor's mitochondria. The healthy donor's egg is pierced and the jelly-like cytoplasm containing hundreds of healthy (at least more healthy) mitochondria is transplanted into the unhealthy embryo. Voila! A 33% increase in survival! Here modern medicine is treating the mitochondrial defect directly by adding new genes into the cells. Little research has been conducted to show what might occur if these mothers were simply given thyroid hormone to increase the number and activity of their own mitochondria, not to mention all of the other benefits that thyroid hormones would offer. My infertility patients usually conceive within months of beginning desiccated thyroid.

In my experience, hypothyroid mothers properly treated with desiccated thyroid prior to their pregnancies appear to give birth to normal thyroid babies. (The physiological functions of thyroid hormones are listed in Appendix A.)

Administering thyroid hormones to our hypothyroid children would allow for normal development of their central nervous systems (especially the brain), bones, sex glands, and impart a better chance for a healthy life. Giving thyroid medicine to hypothyroid adults would drastically reduce many chronic illnesses, premature deaths, and suffering. Properly functioning mitochondria would allow the other 46 chromosomes that delineate our individuality to fully express themselves in a healthy and dynamic cellular environment.

A growing number of advanced medical scientists now understand the importance of the genetic changes in mito-chondria. A groundswell of environmental medicine doctors and scientists are recognizing that pervasive environmental toxins are disrupting thyroid and other hormonal functions. However, the fact that this combination of genetics and toxins results in hypothyroidism remains unknown. Chapter 12 will elucidate the deleterious impact of environmental toxins.

I propose this mitochondria based illness be called Type 2 hypothyroidism. It results in exactly the same symptoms, physical findings, and disease processes as primary failure of the thyroid gland, which should be termed Type 1 hypothyroidism.

Additional Genetic Causes

Type 2 hypothyroidism is not simply due to mitochondrial mutations. There also are a whole set of other inherited disorders already described in modern textbooks on hypothyroidism. These are the dominant and recessive single gene patterns termed "Mendelian." These traits are passed through our set of 46 chromosomes and may be contributed by one or both parents. Therefore, either parent may contribute faulty genes resulting in Type 2 hypothyroidism.

There are receptors for thyroid hormones both on the surface and within every cell. Around one hundred different mutations have been found in one of the primary genes for thyroid receptors.[35] Defective thyroid receptors may prevent a sufficient supply of hormones that are circulating in our blood from reaching the mitochondria and other crucial sites such as the nucleus of the cell. The nucleus is where the thyroid hormones activate genes and stimulate protein synthesis, among a host of other tasks. Refer to Appendix A for details on the effects of thyroid hormones. All of these vital physiological mechanisms may be affected.

Numerous steps are involved in the synthesis of thyroid hormones, their storage, secretion, delivery, and utilization. All of these vital physiological mechanisms may be affected.

Enzymes are protein molecules that catalyze (speed up or facilitate) chemical reactions of other substances. The chemical reactions that transform thyroid hormones into energy require a milieu of enzymes and coenzymes. Coenzymes are an organic nonprotein molecule that binds with a protein molecule to form the active enzyme. Partial or complete blockage of any of these steps from genetic defects or environmental toxins may result in Type 2 hypothyroidism.[93,95] Environmental toxins interfere with all aspects of normal cellular functions. The impact these toxins have on our increasingly susceptible population is profound. Chapter 12 will highlight the environmental health disaster that is upon us. Appendix B lists the synthetic chemicals known to interfere with the production, transport, and metabolism of thyroid hormones. The next chapter will show us how our medical establishment became enamored with blood tests in their attempts to diagnose hypothyroidism.

Chemicals, Pollutants, and Pesticides
In Umbilical Cord Blood

A 2004 U.S. study revealed that pregnant women's umbilical cord blood is contaminated with an average of 200 industrial chemicals and pollutants. Of the 287 chemicals detected, 180 are known to cause cancer in humans or animals, 217 are toxic to the brain and nervous system, and 208 cause birth defects or abnormal development in animals (www.ewg.org).[102]

Our unborn children are bathed in a toxic womb. Chapter 12 illustrates how these pollutants create far reaching effects upon the thyroid hormones.

Chapter 7
Laboratory Tests for Hypothyroidism

Why does your doctor insist that you can't possibly suffer from hypothyroidism if your lab tests are normal?

Remember an earlier statement I made: Hypothyroidism was formerly considered difficult to diagnose due to the insidious nature of onset and the myriad paradoxical symptoms it may produce. For years after the discovery of hypothyroidism, its diagnosis depended upon the doctors' ability to ask the right questions and look for the most common physical findings associated with the disease.

Use of the basal metabolic rate (BMR) test began early in the twentieth century to aid doctors' decision-making process. Doctors were frequently led astray by the inaccuracies of the test. However, many doctors were aware of the test's fallibility and would give patients suspected of having hypothyroidism a trial of thyroid hormones despite a normal BMR (refer to the Basal Metabolism section in Chapter 1).

The ultimate test of whether or not a patient was hypothyroid was the patient's response to a trial of thyroid hormones. Confirmation depended upon improvement or resolution of their symptoms.

The quest for a more accurate test continued throughout the twentieth century. The list of thyroid blood tests grew until there were scores of available tests. Unfortunately, they failed to improve the ability to detect Type 2 hypothyroidism.

Today, the overwhelming majority of doctors are taught to check only the patients' blood tests if they suspect hypothyroidism. If the tests are normal, the search begins for other possible causes of their problems.

The vast majority of patients with hypothyroidism have normal thyroid blood tests, because the tests do not detect Type 2 hypothyroidism. Countless new syndromes, both mental and physical, have been adopted in attempts to explain the myriad symptoms related to hypothyroidism.

The first blood test purported to test thyroid function was introduced in the 1940s. It was the protein-bound iodine test or PBI. Thyroid hormones contain lots of iodine. The PBI test measured the total amount of iodine molecules circulating in blood, which were bound to protein molecules.

It was meant to reflect the total amount of thyroid hormone in the blood. It turned out that the test also detected iodine in the diet, such as iodized salt. There were other problems with the test as well.

The PBI was initially touted to be the answer to doctors' difficulties regarding the often subtle and troublesome diagnosis. A 1954 monograph in *American Lectures in Endocrinology* entitled "Hypothyroidism, an Essay on Modern Medicine" devoted 26 pages to the intricacies of the PBI. The author was Chairman of the Department of Medicine from the University of Southern California. In it, he stated, "The diagnosis of hypothyroidism is at present best made by the determination of the protein bound iodine."[37]

Finally, in 1967, a study published in *The Journal of the American Medical Association* put an end to any suggestions regarding the validity of using the PBI to diagnose hypothyroidism.[38] Dr. Barnes, discussing the PBI in his book, stated: "Nevertheless, for many years, some otherwise competent physicians swore by the PBI as an accurate index of thyroid function while the rest of us swore at it."[4]

As late as 1975, "the" leading medical textbook on hypothyroidism, *The Thyroid and Its Diseases,* addressed the confusing array of tests, which were available at the time. I quote from the text under the heading "Thyroid Function Tests-Introduction," "A plethora of thyroid tests are available, and each year new ones appear. Physicians grow used to one examination only to have it replaced by another that allegedly is more specific or useful. There seems to be no easy defense against this 'scientific progress.'" Sixteen different principal diagnostic tests were listed as well as a number of other tests.[39]

There are several physiological assumptions on which the validity of blood tests for hypothyroidism depend (see corresponding numbers in diagram below):

1. The peripheral tissues transmit their need for thyroid hormones to the brain.
2. The part of the brain called the hypothalamus transmits these signals to another part of the brain called the pituitary gland.
3. The pituitary secretes thyroid stimulating hormone (TSH), which gives the signal to the thyroid gland to secrete more thyroid hormones.
4. The thyroid hormones are transported to the peripheral tissues via the blood.
5. The action of the thyroid hormones on the tissues reduces the demand on the brain for more thyroid hormones. More accurately, thyroid hormones are utilized inside each of our cells. The trillions of cells that make up all of our tissues and organs must be able to signal their need for more hormones.

Thyroid Pathways

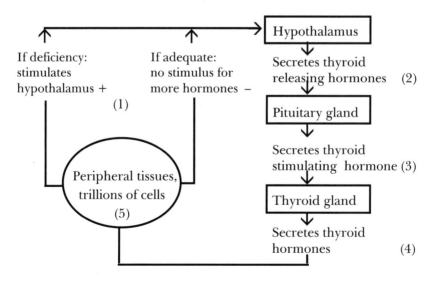

The critical assumption in this fifth step is that our cells are able to transmit their need for thyroid hormones back to the brain. Apparently, this fifth step is where the bulk of the problem occurs. To me, it appears that it is impossible for genetically defective mitochondria in our cells to transmit these signals. None of the expanding volumes of research on patients with defective mitochondria report any unusual deviation from normal regarding the thyroid function blood tests.

A large number of environmental toxins also adversely affect many different steps in the complicated schemata of thyroid hormone metabolism, including impedance or destruction of mitochondrial function. Medical studies at The Environmental Health Center of Dallas have demonstrated resolution of many symptoms of hypothyroidism including subnormal basal temperatures after the patients underwent detoxification. The vast majority of these patients also had normal thyroid test results before and after undergoing detoxification. **Therefore, the environmental toxins' impact also escapes the paradigm that doctors have relied upon for decades. As you will see, Chapter 12 is devoted to the growing threat of environmental toxins that disrupt our thyroid metabolism.**[40,41,42]

The thyroid stimulating hormone (TSH) blood test was introduced commercially in the late 1960s. By no means did the TSH receive a glowing review in *The Thyroid and Its Diseases*, the preeminent medical textbook from 1975. On the contrary, numerous problems were discussed.[39]

The thyroid stimulating hormone, or TSH, was determined to have a normal range through a series of blood tests on a large number of people. There are three possible test results for the TSH: high, low, or normal. Many doctors continue to debate the "normal" range, which has changed on several occasions.

If the TSH is high or above the normal range, doctors interpret that to mean the body's cells are telling the brain they need more thyroid hormone. The relay system in the brain is trying to stimulate production of more thyroid hormones. Hence, the patient with a high level of thyroid stimulating hormone (TSH) is deemed hypothyroid.

When the TSH test is below "normal," the interpretation is the thyroid gland is producing too many thyroid hormones. The body's cells are telling the brain to decrease thyroid hormone production by decreasing thyroid stimulating hormone (TSH). If the TSH test were infallible, patients with a TSH that is below normal (suppressed) would be <u>hyper</u>thyroid. In other words, their thyroid would be producing too many hormones and the feedback mechanism to reduce the production of thyroid hormones has begun. However, the TSH is more than occasionally low in "normal" patients. It is a far cry from being infallible. Additional different thyroid tests are required to prove a patient is <u>hyper</u>thyroid when a low TSH is present.

> Modern medicine has adopted the TSH as the "GOLD STANDARD." If the TSH is normal, the search for hypothyroidism usually ends.

The section following the TSH discussion in *The Thyroid and Its Diseases* addressed the basal metabolic rate (BMR). Problems associated with obtaining an accurate BMR are mentioned. However, at the end of the text's discussion on BMR, the authors stated, "It is the only available test that reflects the metabolic rate of the whole organism, and measures directly thyroid hormone activity at the tissue level. In this regard it is in contrast to most other measurements, which are one or two steps removed from the final target site."[39]

So how did doctors become so convinced of the invincibility of the TSH? It is a confusing trail at best. A prominent medical textbook on hypothyroidism was published in 2000. *Warner & Ingbar's The Thyroid: A Fundamental and Clinical Text*, devotes a chapter to the TSH, other thyroid hormone measurements, and their relative importance. I quote the first paragraph: "The single best test for assessment of thyroid function is measurement of serum thyrotropin (TSH). That is because assays for serum TSH are highly sensitive in detecting either thyrotoxicosis or primary hypothyroidism" (thyrotoxicosis is <u>hyper</u>thyroidism).[11]

Absolutely **no references** are given to prove the validity of this statement. This is the medical dogma of our time.

From the same paragraph, "TSH screening of all women over 50 years of age is now recommended by The American College of Physicians. Women over 50 are thought to be at highest risk. **The screening is necessary because repeated studies have shown doctors, including endocrinologists, are not capable of making the diagnosis of hypothyroidism from the patients' histories and physical exams.**"[11] This further illustrates how doctors have come to rely almost solely on the results of laboratory tests to make their diagnosis for them.

To cite an example: A 1988 Swedish study, referenced in this same chapter, reported primary care doctors in one clinic screened 2,000 consecutive adult patients for hypothyroidism. Following the history and physical exam, the doctors suspected 35 patients were suffering the illness. Unfortunately, none of the 35 patients had an elevated TSH. Therefore, the doctors concluded that their patients could not have hypothyroidism.

In addition, 21 other patients in the study were diagnosed with hypothyroidism from abnormal TSH values. None of these patients were suspected of having thyroid disease after the initial history and physical exam. Therefore, the researchers recommended that all patients be screened.[43]

Another Scandinavian study touted by the same text demonstrated the need to screen all patients' thyroid blood tests. Three endocrinologists separately examined 55 consecutive patients referred to their clinic because of suspected thyroid disease. Following the history and physical exam, the three doctors' diagnoses were in agreement in only 55% of the patients. When blood tests, including the TSH, were added, they agreed about

90% of the time. **Somehow, the thyroid blood tests were deemed more reliable than the patients' histories and physical exams.**[44]

The TSH is the problem. It only detects a small fraction of hypothyroidism. WHY?

The studies, which Drs. Barnes, Sonkin, Hertoghe, and I performed, clearly showed patients with normal blood tests, including the TSH, suffered all the manifestations of hypothyroidism. They had low basal metabolism tests, low basal temperatures, and most importantly, their symptoms improved or resolved when given thyroid hormones.

Therefore, the problem is exactly where Drs. Barnes and Sonkin said it was, inside each cell where thyroid hormones perform their work. The inherited cellular defects in mitochondria, as well as synthetic toxins, impair thyroid hormone metabolism at the cellular level. These cellular problems somehow avoid the schemata of our intricate feedback mechanism necessary to maintain adequate thyroid function. Despite normal levels of TSH and thyroid hormones in the bloodstream, patients with Type 2 hypothyroidism require additional thyroid hormones to overcome their defective cellular metabolism.

I wondered how mainstream medicine went so far astray? I hoped *The Textbook of Medical Physiology* might provide the answer. Unfortunately, it did not. The section entitled, "Regulation of Thyroid Hormone Secretion" goes into great detail. From the first paragraph under this topic, "To maintain a normal basal metabolic rate, precisely the right amount of thyroid hormone must be secreted all the time, and, to provide this, a specific feedback mechanism operates through the hypothalamus and anterior pituitary gland to control the rate of thyroid secretion."[33] The hypothalamus and pituitary glands are located in our brains and are integral components of the endocrine system. No references are given, no basal metabolism studies to back up the statement, absolutely nothing. **The blind assumption that our bodies' intricate hormone regulation system is infallible remains the paramount mistake in the practice of modern medicine.**

I am intentionally being redundant in order to establish one crucial fact. There is no scientific evidence to support the doctors' claim that the TSH test detects hypothyroidism in the vast majority of patients. The validity of the TSH has been established by word of mouth and purportedly by the studies I have presented.

In 1997, a group of endocrinologists attempted to correlate the classical symptoms and physical findings associated with hypothyroidism with modern thyroid blood tests. This was the first study in almost 30 years in which doctors attempted to demonstrate the clinical efficacy of the thyroid function blood tests. It was published in *The Journal of Clinical Endocrinology*.[45] Despite being mired in the myriad sophisticated thyroid blood tests and lacking clinical trials of giving thyroid hormones to symptomatic patients with normal blood tests, a very revealing conclusion was reached:

"It is of special interest that some patients with severe biochemical hypothyroidism had only mild clinical signs, whereas other patients with minor biochemical changes had quite severe clinical manifestations. Thus, we assume that tissue hypothyroidism at the peripheral target organs must be different in an individual patient. Therefore, the clinical score can give a valuable estimate of the individual severity of metabolic hypothyroidism."[45] This is an excellent illustration of Type 2 hypothyroidism without the authors even knowing it.

In other words, there frequently is no correlation between the blood tests for hypothyroidism and the severity of the disease. Despite this conclusion, the authors would not endorse their new clinical score for diagnosing hypothyroidism.

They selected 50 female patients with "overt" hypothyroidism. Their "overtness" was based on elevated TSH tests. Eighty "normal" women were used to compare the frequency of hypothyroid symptoms both groups shared. The 80 women were normal because their TSH was normal. This group also passed a basic physical exam.

Can you guess why the authors would not endorse using the classical symptoms of hypothyroidism to help doctors with the diagnosis? There were too many overlapping symptoms between the two groups. The authors stated, "In the control group [the normal group], older women presented more often with hypothyroid symptoms, especially constipation and dry skin, compared with younger controls."[45] Remember that women over 50 are at highest risk. The authors would never consider that there might be a problem with the thyroid function blood tests. To eliminate this problem, the scores were "adjusted" for age. Women younger than 55 had their scores weighted more heavily than their older counterparts.

Also, for the new scoring system to be meaningful, cold intolerance (feeling cold easily) and a slow pulse rate had to be eliminated altogether. Too many "normal" women demonstrated these classical symptoms of hypothyroidism. Therefore, the authors' new "adjusted" clinical scores were recommended for use only if coupled with thyroid blood tests to assess individual assessment of thyroid failure and to monitor treatment.

The authors are blinded by their devotion to the laboratory tests. A large percentage of the "normals" no doubt suffered Type 2 hypothyroidism. This study also received prominent mention in the latest text on hypothyroidism, *Warner & Ingbar's The Thyroid: A Fundamental and Clinical Text*. It purportedly provided further evidence of the infallibility of our technologically advanced thyroid blood tests.

Patients would have been much better off if doctors stuck with the basal metabolism test. Dr. Barnes' studies demonstrated the superior efficacy of the basal temperature test, which never came into vogue.

The Hertoghe's endocrinology clinic and doctors at the Central Laboratory in Antwerp, Belgium developed a reliable urine test for hypothyroidism in 1984. The test reflects how the body utilizes the thyroid hormones, not their mere presence in the blood. Urine is collected over a 24-hour period. T3 thyroid hormones in the urine are measured and give an accurate assessment of an individual's thyroid function.[46] Unfortunately, the Hertoghe's method of measuring the amount of T3 hormone has not been standardized and may be difficult to reproduce in other laboratories. The Barnes Foundation recommends it. More details about the test will be discussed in Chapter 9.

A significant autopsy study from 1992 found that the patients' medical histories led to the correct final diagnosis in 76% of cases, the physical exam in 12%, and the laboratory investigations in 11%.[47]

Doctors currently ignore patients' medical histories and physical findings consistent with hypothyroidism. The laboratory tests for the illness reign supreme.

With respect to hypothyroidism, several generations of primary care physicians and endocrinologists have been trained to treat blood tests and not patients. Specialists and primary doctors no longer ask the proper questions or look for the telltale physical findings that make the diagnosis obvious.

During the 1990s, Dr. Sonkin particularly opposed a new method of treating hypothyroidism advocated by a prominent group of doctors. He referred to them as the "Fine Tuners". Their theory was to control the latest "ultra-sensitive" TSH blood test within a very narrow range. The narrow range theoretically was the ideal "physiological" or normal range. Several new strengths of synthetic thyroid dosages were produced in order to satisfy the need to precisely manipulate the TSH. There was never any mention of the patients' symptoms or physical findings in the Fine Tuners' literature. Their method became widely accepted.

I also witnessed the negative consequences that resulted from the Fine Tuners. One of my former patients is an ideal representation. A charming 87 year-old patient entered my office using a cane, bent at the waist and in great distress from pain. The patient had been to numerous physicians whose opinions all favored back surgery. The patient's daughter was a nurse and aware of my practice.

My thorough history revealed her pain was related to hormones. Eleven months earlier, a physician tested her TSH and found it "suppressed" or lower than normal. The woman had been taking the same dosage of thyroid hormones as long as she could remember (decades). To the physician, Fine Tuner, this meant an immediate reduction in thyroid hormones was necessary. At that time, the widowed 87 year-old patient's life was full of vigor with regular dances and a job taking care of younger women.

Her pain began gradually within several months of the reduced thyroid dosage and became disabling within six months. She could no longer drive, dance, take care of herself, and was in constant pain. Not one of the physicians thought to ask about her long-standing hypothyroidism. After restoring her dosage to the previous level and treating her sore muscles, she resumed dancing, gardening, and taking care of younger women.

Endocrinologists from my town were no exception, as they relied on blood tests to make the diagnosis of hypothyroidism for them. One endocrinologist in particular appeared to suffer from an advanced case of Type 2 hypothyroidism upon first glance. **"The general uniformity of the more prominent symptoms is, indeed, remarkable, allowing ready recognition of the malady in any freshly encountered case by an observer who has seen one well pronounced case"** (from the initial British summary in 1888).[1] Their 200 page summary of hypothyroidism was the first comprehensive report on the illness.

The following illustrations were used to demonstrate the features of the illness from the original reports in 1888 (no ages given).

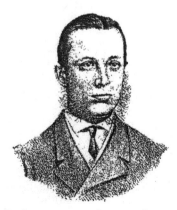
Before onset of myxedema

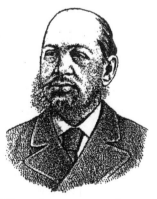
Myxedema, years later

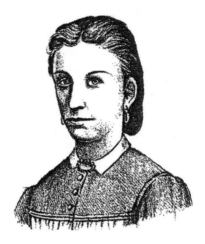

Before myxedema
age 21

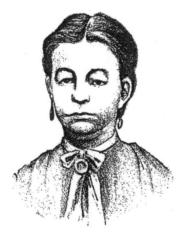

Mild myxedema
age 28

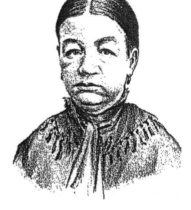

Marked myxedema
age 32

Source: Clinical Society of London. 1888. *Report of The Committee of The Clinical Society of London to Investigate the Subject of Myxoedema. Transactions Clinical Society London.* Supp. Vol. 21. London: Clinical Society of London.

How many of your family members and friends bear a resemblance to these pictures? Being overweight is not a prerequisite for hypothyroidism to be present. Large percentages are of normal height and weight. Often, many of the most advanced cases suffer wasting symptoms, if they live long enough.

Reliance on blood tests to both diagnose and treat hypothyroidism, combined with the use of synthetic thyroid hormones instead of desiccated thyroid, no longer produces the striking resolution of myxedema or the transformation of physical features pictured in older textbooks. Pictures of hypothyroid patients before treatment with thyroid hormones, and follow-up pictures after treatment, have disappeared from medical textbooks published during the last 40 years.

One of the last texts to include such pictures was the *Atlas of Clinical Endocrinology* published in 1957 by Roberto Escamilla M.D., and H. Lisser, M.D., who was the former President of The Endocrine Society and Clinical Professor Emeritus of Medicine and Endocrinology from the University of California. This text included dozens of helpful photographs and case studies ranging from infants to the elderly.[48]

The following pictures show the resolution of myxedema in a man, aged 51, over an 18 month period of treatment. He suffered muscle soreness and stiffness, constipation, cold intolerance, cholesterol level 277, and basal metabolic rate (BMR) of minus 37% before treatment with desiccated thyroid hormones.

Figure 1a. 51 year-old man formerly sang tenor, now sings bass. BMR was minus 37%, cholesterol 277 mg percent. He suffered muscular soreness and stiffness, constipation, and cold intolerance.

Figure 1b. Three months after treatment, BMR was minus 2.5%. Again sings tenor.

Figure 1c. Same patient after 1 1/2 years treatment.

Fig. 1a   Fig. 1b   Fig. 1c

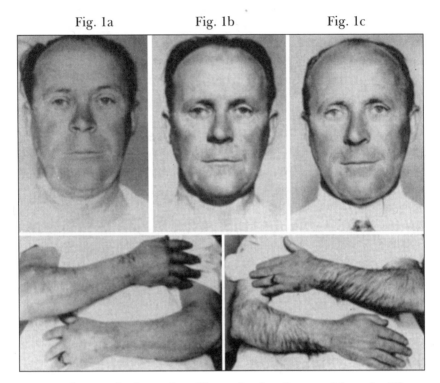

Note the resolution of puffiness in the face and hands. The hair on his arms evolved from scant, coarse, and brittle into long, soft, and luxurious.

Source: Lisser, H., and Escamilla, R. F. *Atlas of Clinical Endocrinology: Including Text of Diagnosis and Treatment.* C.V. Mosby Company, 1957. Reprinted with permission.

Numerous senior citizens have relayed to me that every time they changed physicians or one retired or died, their dosage of thyroid replacement was decreased or discontinued. Consequently, they were not just suffering from chronic pain but numerous other symptoms of hypothyroidism.

How many patients have heard this from their doctors? **"You will have heart trouble and develop osteoporosis if you take thyroid medication when the TSH is normal."** Unfortunately, many of my patients were told this erroneous warning, and a large percentage never returned for treatment. They were informed by their doctors that their normal TSH test precluded any chance of being hypothyroid. The logic being, if they were to take the thyroid hormones I recommended, they would become hyperthyroid. However, as the studies have shown, they would not.

Dr. Barnes' studies demonstrated proper treatment of hypothyroidism actually protected against heart attacks (Chapter 3). Dr. Zondek was the first of many doctors to demonstrate resolution of congestive heart failure (CHF) after treatment with thyroid hormones. Zondek's study was published in 1918. X-rays showing resolution of his patient's heart failure are included in a section devoted to the heart in Chapter 8.[31] Doctors have long known both hypothyroidism and hyperthyroidism cause problems with our hearts and bones. Osteoporosis may result from either.

Bones may become abnormally thickened and their infra-structure weakened due to hypothyroidism. After the patient is placed on thyroid hormones, the bones begin to remodel. Stronger, thinner bones gradually replace the weak infrastructure. The remodeling process may take as long as 6 to 12 months after an adequate dosage of thyroid hormones is given. It may take several months to reach this dosage.

Two clinical studies, which supposedly proved that suppressing the TSH caused bone loss (osteoporosis), were published in 1988 and 1991. In both studies, premenopausal women were chosen to eliminate the increased risk all women have of osteoporosis after menopause. Bone density studies were performed on women with no history of thyroid disease and were compared to studies on age-matched women with a history of thyroid illnesses.[49,50] The women with histories of thyroid illnesses had been on enough levothyroxine (T4) to keep their TSH blood tests below the normal range for at least five years. According to the TSH dogma, these women were presumed to be "subclinically" hyperthyroid. The subclinical term is due to the fact that they did not have any symptoms of hyperthyroidism. The women with low TSH tests had more osteoporosis than the women with no history of thyroid related illnesses.

Bone density studies were done only once, at the time of the comparison. The bone densities of the women with prior histories of thyroid disease never had been previously tested. These women remained hypothyroid in spite of treatment with T4 and low TSH test results. Their hypothyroidism predisposed them toward having osteoporosis. As I will discuss in the chapter devoted to treatment, the synthetic thyroid hormone, T4 (Synthroid®, levothyroxine, etc.), has never been proven to resolve the symptoms of hypothyroidism in long-term clinical trials.

Also, in the one bone density study where the dosages of levothyroxine (T4) were given, 27 out of the 28 patients were receiving between .1 and .2 mg daily. My patients were receiving these same dosages when they came to me for help. A list of patients' symptoms that were already being treated for hypothyroidism when they came to me for help is included in the next section of this chapter. I wonder how the symptom list from the women in the two bone density studies would compare with the symptoms my patients suffered. However, there was no mention of symptoms in either major research study.

The following studies in clinical journals stated that suppressing the TSH did not cause bone loss.[51,52,53] However, the conclusions from the initial studies persist. Forty percent of elderly American women suffer osteoporosis. This percentage is equal to the number of Americans Dr. Barnes stated were hypothyroid in 1976. The incidence will not decline until Type 2 hypothyroidism is recognized and treated.

One of my patients in Missouri expressed concern about being <u>hyper</u>thyroid. Another doctor discovered his TSH was very low and apprised him of his supposedly dire prognosis. My patient wasted little time calling my office in Georgia. The patient had previously suffered severe depression, chronic pain, high cholesterol, and other symptoms of hypothyroidism, most of which had long since resolved. He had taken the 3 grains of desiccated thyroid I prescribed for years. I asked my patient if he had any signs of <u>hyper</u>thyroidism such as a rapid heartbeat, palpitations, constant sweating, weight loss, weakness, frequent stools, increased tremor, or if his basal temperature had suddenly risen from its usual 97 degrees to above 98.2 °F? "No, nothing like that," was his response. He had internal hemorrhoids and some blood in his stool. Otherwise, he was doing just fine. There were no symptoms of <u>hyper</u>thyroidism. He checked his basal temperature again to reassure himself.

Oral desiccated thyroid was the "standard of care" for 80 years. The dosages prescribed were several times larger than dosages used since the 1970s. **No cases of osteoporosis or fractures from the usage of the higher dosages were ever reported in the literature.**

My Patients

In 1998, I decided to review my pain patients' medical histories, symptoms, and physical findings after realizing the pervasiveness of Type 2 hypothyroidism. Random chart reviews were performed on 162 adult patients out of over 500 patients. Most of these patients were seen prior to my discovering the Barnes Foundation. Therefore, the results no doubt would have been higher in a number of categories had I been aware of all the symptoms attributable to hypothyroidism.

The metamorphosis of my history taking and physical exam took place over a period of years. The questions I asked changed, as did the subtleties I looked for on physical exam. For instance, cold hands (often with clammy palms) and cold flat feet would have scored much higher had I begun looking for them sooner. Weakness is one of the most common symptoms of hypothyroidism. Unfortunately, I did not distinguish between weakness and fatigue.

Here is the listing of symptoms from my 162 chart reviews, which included 118 females and 44 males. The average age was 49 years in both groups. I also separated 34 patients who were already being treated for hypothyroidism out of the 162.

Six patients had been referred to me who had no pain, hence, the 96% figure under the listing of "pain" in the following chart reviews. Pain is merely one symptom of a much larger problem. Pain need not be present in a hypothyroid person. One old study from Dr. Ian Ramsey's book, *Thyroid Disease and Muscle Dysfunction*, estimated that around 50% of patients suffering the illness complained of pain.[36]

Table 7.1   **Starr Pain Clinic Patients: 162 Chart Reviews**

	Number of Patients	Percentage
Pain	156	96
Dry Skin	137	85
Fatigue	134	83
Brittle/Ridged Nails	131	81
Menstrual problems (females)	81	69
Depression	91	57
Myxedema:		
Moderate to Marked	88	54
Cold Intolerance	86	53
Insomnia	86	53
Delayed Ankle Reflexes	80	49
Hysterectomy (females)	48	41
Allergies	66	41
Cold Hands or Feet	62	38
Weight Gain	61	38
Constipation	52	32
High Blood Pressure	50	31
Tension (anxiety)	47	29
Headaches	46	28
Hair Loss	45	28
TMJ-Teeth Clenching	40	25
Paresthesias (tingling)	38	24
Hypothyroidism, Type 1	34	21
Tremor	31	19
Heart Disease	27	17
Diabetes	26	16
Heat Intolerance	25	15
Cancer	15	9
Autoimmune Disease	12	7
Hypoglycemia	11	7
Emphysema	8	5

Table 7.2   **Starr Pain Clinic Patients with
Prior Diagnosis of Hypothyroidism**

Already receiving treatment (T4, i.e. levothyroxine), dosage
range 0.1 mg (100 mcg) to 0.2 mg (200 mcg) per day.

	Number of Patients	Percentage
Hypothyroidism Type 1	34	100
Dry Skin	29	85
Fatigue	29	85
Brittle/Ridged Nails	28	82
Menstrual Problems (females)	20	67
Cold Intolerance	22	65
Depression	20	59
Myxedema:		
Moderate to Marked	19	56
Delayed Ankle Reflexes	19	56
Cold Hands or Feet	17	50
Insomnia	17	50
Hair Loss	16	47
Allergies	15	44
Tension (anxiety)	14	41
Weight Gain	14	41
High Blood Pressure	10	29
Hysterectomy (females)	7	23
Diabetes	9	26
Heat Intolerance	9	26
Paresthesias (tingling)	9	26
Tremor	7	21
Constipation	7	21
TMJ-Teeth Clenching	7	21
Headaches	6	18
Heart Disease	5	15
Cancer	4	12
Emphysema	3	9

The patients who were already being treated for Type 1 hypothyroidism continued to suffer as many symptoms as the untreated group of patients with Type 2 hypothyroidism. In my opinion, the Type 1 patients already receiving treatment suffered from both Type 1 and Type 2 hypothyroidism. Their family histories left no doubt in my mind this was indeed the case. Recall endocrine glands such as the thyroid are prominently affected by declines in cellular energy. Judging from the Type 1 patients' constellation of symptoms, the treatment they were receiving was woefully lacking. Many of these patients' symptoms resolved with additional thyroid hormone treatment.

In Chapter 9 under Treatment Guidelines, I present a similar, much larger study authored by Dr. Jacques Hertoghe (the third generation Belgian endocrinologist) that confirms these findings.

Over half of my patients had moderate to marked myxedema on physical exam, the telltale sign of hypothyroidism. With few exceptions, the patients I treated since discovering Dr. Barnes' basal temperature test were below 97.8 °F. Their marked myxedema, as well as the constellation of symptomatology consistent with hypothyroidism, should raise many questions. As stated in Chapter 1, a group of 50 consecutive pain patients with normal thyroid (TSH) blood tests averaged 15% below normal basal metabolism. A reading of 10% below normal, coupled with symptoms of hypothyroidism, was formerly considered strongly indicative of the disease (see Basal Metabolism, Chapter 1).

My chart reviews represent the suffering of a minute portion of the affected population in a relatively small town. I now practice medicine in a much larger city. The prevalence of Type 1 and Type 2 hypothyroidism and the resultant suffering among my new patients has not changed.

Modern doctors use the thyroid blood tests as guidelines for treatment as well as diagnosis. The end result is the health disaster that is upon us. Chapter 9 is devoted to the successful treatment of hypothyroidism.

Chapter 8
Symptoms of Type 1 and 2 Hypothyroidism

Introduction

Eugene Hertoghe M.D., began his work in the late nineteenth century and devoted much of his energy to the study of hypothyroidism. Dr. Hertoghe was the first doctor to recognize the prevalence of mild forms of the illness. He traveled to America and addressed The International Surgical Congress at the New York Polyclinic School and Hospital in 1914. There, he summarized the ramifications of hypothyroidism eloquently, "We know that without the thyroid stimulus no cell, whatever it may be, can attain its morphological perfection—the perfection needed for good work, muscular, nervous, connective, glandular, or bone."[32]

As previously stated, a textbook authored by a renowned German doctor, Hermann Zondek, *Diseases of the Endocrine Glands*, was published in German in 1926 and reprinted in English in 1944. This text was meant to aid doctors with the diagnosis and treatment of hypothyroidism and other hormone problems.

Drs. Hertoghe and Zondek described numerous symptoms and physical characteristics of hypothyroidism, many of which have vanished from today's textbooks. From Dr. Zondek's book, "**The signs observed more or less regularly are: General indolence and inertia, lassitude, constipation, anorexia, tendency to fat deposits especially around the hips and above the mons veneris [the pubic bone], deep depression of the root of the nose, delayed dentition and caries [tooth decay], chilly sensation, dry skin, swelling and pallor [paleness] of the mucous membranes, enlarged tongue, rheumatoid pains, sometimes in the joints, oppressive feelings and convulsive pains in the cardiac region. Skeletal changes are common, particularly scoliosis and general contraction of the pelvis. Chronic deforming changes in the joints are observed.**"[8]

Hypothyroidism is much more easily treated in young, relatively healthy patients, before the disease is firmly established and has wrought all of its mental and physical infirmities. However, proper treatment of Type 1 and Type 2 hypothyroidism can produce dramatic results no matter what the patient's age.

Prior to the twentieth century, many more women than men suffered hypothyroidism. The reason may have been the tremendous hormonal stresses associated with monthly menstrual cycles, pregnancies, and menopause. Dr. Zondek stated there is a great want of thyroid hormone during the menses and only then may symptoms be apparent. Today, the incidence in men is fast approaching that in women, due to the plague of environmental toxins affecting our thyroid metabolism coupled with the fact that modern medicine has enabled several generations to survive and pass on deleterious genes.

Infants and Children

Susceptibility to infection has always been one of the cardinal signs of hypothyroidism. The upper respiratory tract, particularly the ears, sinuses, throat, and lungs is a common target. The urinary tract also is a frequent target. Resistance against viral diseases and fungal infections such as yeast is low among the hypothyroid. In The National Institutes of Health study involving over 100 patients with known genetically inherited hypothyroidism, 56% had frequent ear, nose, and throat infections.[35]

Any organ system may be involved. Every cell between and including the **hair** on the head and the **toenails** (both of which are frequently affected) depends upon proper thyroid function for development and health. Thin and/or dry hair are possible symptoms. Redheads have a particularly high incidence of hypothyroidism. Healthy toenails have pink nail beds and are hard. Many children I have examined have cold, flat feet, pale nail beds, or ridged, striated, and soft nails. Two reasons for this are that circulation and the synthesis of new proteins are impaired (see Appendix A).

If we consider that Type 2 hypothyroidism is usually present from birth, then the illness is in many ways comparable to the congenital or endemic cretinism of old. **Dr. Zondek emphasized disturbances of growth, anomalies in genital development, and signs of mental disturbance as "the factors whose development is chiefly governed by the thyroid gland."**[8] Therefore, let us first consider current trends in growth, genital development, and mentation among our children.

Growth Disturbances

Thyroid hormones are a powerful stimulus for growth and development of bones. Textbooks are replete with literature about hypothyroidism resulting in short stature. The fact that accelerated growth and tall stature is also characteristic of the illness is less well known. I have noted hypothyroidism in my tall patients and friends. I cannot help notice a number of obviously hypothyroid mothers. They often have very tall daughters with narrow hips (contraction of the pelvis). In Dr. Barnes' research, people over six feet tall consistently ran slightly lower than normal basal temperatures and suffered varying degrees of hypothyroidism.[22] Dr. Barnes stated, "On the one hand, a marked deficiency occurring at an early age may lead to growth failure and dwarfism, a minor deficiency not only may allow growth to proceed at a normal rate, but to be accelerated and extended, producing a seven footer."[4]

The average size of Americans has literally ballooned in the last 30 years. As an old Missouri football player commented, "The tremendous size of today's players is just not right." The average men's shoe size has gone from a size 9 in the 1970s to an 11 today. Our average height increased several inches during the twentieth century and obesity is pervasive. The opposite may also occur. Small stature or short segments in the upper or lower limbs are common anomalies. The arms or legs may appear too short or small for the torso.

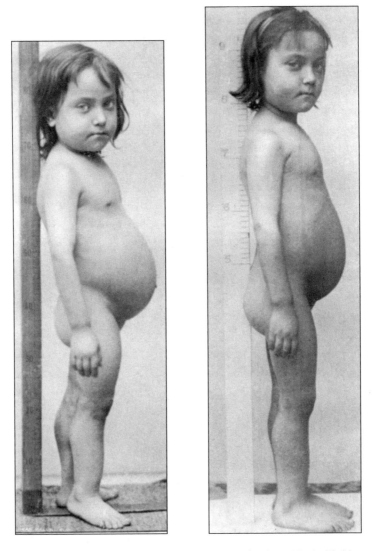

Source: Hertoghe, E. *The Practitioner*, Jan 1915, Vol XCIV, No 1, 26-93.

This seven year-old girl stood 2 feet 11 inches before treatment. Her abdomen was protuberant, and she suffered severe constipation. Her neck was quite short, and the bones in her lower legs bowed outwards. After eight months of treatment with thyroid, she had grown over eight inches, her stomach was receding, and the neck had elongated.[2]

A number of my patients reported birth defects of their joints that required bracing and other corrections in their infancy. The hips and lower extremities were usually involved.

An infant's head may appear disproportionately large and tend to protrude or drop forward. The wide seams of soft tissue that join several of these bones in infants' heads are called "fontanels." The anterior fontanel is the largest and slowest to fuse. It is located on top of the skull toward the front. Normally, it hardens around the middle of the second year. The posterior fontanel normally closes around three months after birth. Hypothyroidism may result in the bones being slow to fuse or join together. The following illustration shows the location of the anterior and posterior fontanels.

Infant Skull

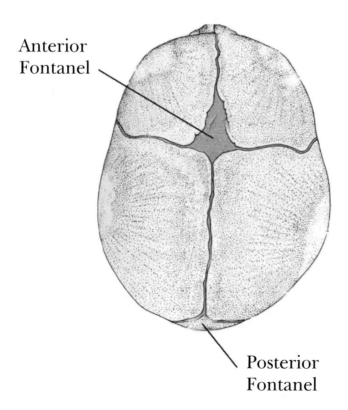

Anterior
Fontanel

Posterior
Fontanel

Recently, I overheard a kind, elderly man politely conversing with a much younger woman. He was explaining how peoples' feet become flatter and wider as their arches gradually fall with age. That statement was true for his generation but is no longer so for our youngsters. Today, many young children suffer flat feet. The lax ligaments that often result from hypothyroidism may not allow the arches to form properly. Normal arch formation proceeds after children are properly treated with thyroid hormones.

Genital Development

Sexual development may be prematurely arrested or precocious (unusually well developed) puberty may result. *Dorland's Medical Dictionary* defines "precocious" to be developed more than is usual at a given age. "Precocity" is defined as "unusually early development of mental or physical traits." These traits are listed in the tables of medical textbooks describing hypothyroidism.

Blacks and other minorities, such as American Indians, are particularly affected with Type 2 hypothyroidism. A recent medical survey of eight year-old children reported 50% of African-American and 15% of whites are now showing signs of puberty. This is indicative of a high incidence of hypothyroidism and reveals why blacks have higher rates of asthma, diabetes, high blood pressure, heart disease, obesity, etc.

Case reports of successful treatment of premature puberty are in the historical literature. If proper treatment with thyroid hormones is given, the pubic hair and secondary sexual characteristics such as breast development disappear. Puberty begins again at age 12 or 13 and progresses normally. Currently, I am treating a 6 year-old for precocious puberty, whose mother has marked myxedema and Type 2 hypothyroidism.

My dear mother was an early developer and had special bathroom privileges at school in the fifth grade. She suffered much of the stigmata associated with hypothyroidism including fatigue, pain, urinary tract infections, hypoglycemia, cold intolerance, dry puffy skin, and developed high blood pressure as well as swelling in her legs as she grew older. I'm happy to say that most of her symptoms resolved with desiccated thyroid therapy.

The incidences of genital deformities are on the rise. The number of males born with hypospadias, where the urethra through which we pass urine opens on the underside of the penis, has climbed markedly in recent years.

Neurological and Mental Problems

Normal function of maternal thyroid is critical for proper brain development of the fetus. Iodine is also crucial (see chapters 9 and 10). Children born to hypothyroid mothers have a higher incidence of visual and spatial processing problems, lowered IQs, and impaired development of many other critical neurological functions.

Dr. Zondek addressed endemic cretinism (infants born with hypothyroidism) in his text. He stated, "The intellect is disturbed in many, but by no means all, patients; the highest degree of idiocy may occur. Very close relations seem to exist between cretinism and deaf-mutism. Very likely both conditions are but different degrees of one disease arising from the same degenerative basis."[8]

Most people with hypothyroidism, including children and adults, tend to be sluggish. However, the illness has paradoxical effects in many different ways. Many children have an abundance of nervous energy or may even be hyperactive.

In a study from the National Institutes of Health published in 1995, attention-deficit hyperactivity disorder (ADHD) was present in 72% of males and 43% of females who were identified with a genetically inherited form of hypothyroidism. The NIH studied 104 affected patients from 42 different families identified between 1976 and 1995. One-third of the affected patients had an IQ of 85 or less.[35]

Medications affecting the central nervous system (the brain and spinal cord) often have the opposite effect upon children than they have on adults. Stimulants such as amphetamines are used to treat hyperactive children with attention deficits. Their hyperactivity and short attention spans frequently improve. These same drugs would make adults more active with shorter attention spans.

The short attention span and hyperactivity many children suffer may be due to their low metabolism and fatigue. If symptoms of hypothyroidism and low basal temperature are present, a trial of thyroid hormones is indicated. Thyroid hormone treatment to increase metabolism is a much more physiological and efficacious method than elevating metabolism with amphetamines.

Dr. Barnes stated, "In the preschool child the history and the basal temperature must make the diagnosis. Most of these children with low thyroid function will have a dull, apathetic appearance and be less active than normal youngsters; yet, here a paradox appears. A few will be nervous, hyperactive and unusually aggressive; emotional problems are frequent. They may cry for no apparent reason and object strenuously to any restrictions. Temper tantrums are common, probably related to undue fatigue. Such youngsters may sleep longer than others and be slow starters in the morning. Their attention span is short; they flit from one activity to another, without becoming engrossed in anything. They adjust poorly to family routines. Frequent infections anywhere in the body are almost pathognomonic [diagnostic] of hypothyroidism."[22] Dr. Barnes also noted that nightmares, as well as other mental aberrations in children, are often resolved with thyroid treatment.[4] Today, 30 years after Dr. Barnes' book was published, a growing percentage of our children suffer early morning fatigue, problems with concentration, and hyperactivity.

Doctors of environmental medicine are churning out reams of successful case reports regarding the treatment of hyperactivity. Children with Type 2 hypothyroidism are much more susceptible to environmental toxins and often suffer from a plethora of allergies and chemical sensitivities.

Childhood depression is rampant and, as previously mentioned, a cardinal sign of hypothyroidism. Manic depression (bipolar disorder) now has its peak onset in the late teens. One generation ago, the peak was in the early 30s. It is occasionally diagnosed in children who demonstrate extreme rage among other symptoms. Both maladies run in families, as does hypothyroidism.

The gray matter of our brain's frontal cortex continues to thicken and grow throughout childhood. Its size peaks at about the time of puberty. It appears the brain has some capacity for regeneration and development throughout our lives. The gray matter of the frontal cortex is involved in judgment, organization, planning, initiating attention, and shifting or stopping attention. The frontal cortex is the command center of the brain.

In 2006, 2.5 million children in America were prescribed antipsychotic medication (www.ahrp.org). Obviously, the earlier the treatment for hypothyroidism begins, the better the chances are for normal cognitive development and psychological well-being.

Other Symptoms

Premature births resulting in small babies, or just the opposite, **long gestations** resulting in large babies, similar to those frequently born to diabetics, may occur. Even with normal gestations, many of the hypothyroid females I have treated had babies in excess of nine pounds prior to beginning thyroid hormones. None imagined that it was a red flag for an insidious illness that was being passed from mother to child. Babies born with developmental defects are also suspect.

Jaundice may appear shortly after birth because of an immature liver. Nasal congestion, noisy breathing, or the tendency to be quiet or sleep more than other babies are signs. A short neck, large head, and a puffy face are possible physical features of the illness.

I knew that a **deep furrowed nose** (usually an indentation or in others, a broad flat area were the nose joins to the face between the eyes) was a developmental abnormality attributable to hypothyroidism. I finally found the reason when I read Dr. Zondek's text. "Faulty growth of the sphenoid bone [a skull bone] is the cause of the characteristic depression of the root of the nose." This gives the face its typical cretinoid appearance. **Deep-set eyes** frequently accompany the furrowed nose. In some cases where myxedema is severe, the face can appear broader than normal and rarely change expression. The expressionless face in severely hypothyroid patients is called "the mask-like face".

The following pictures illustrate the appearance of a 9 month-old hypothyroid infant. She was followed for 21 months after initiating treatment with desiccated thyroid hormones.

Fig. 1a   Fig. 1b   Fig. 1c   Fig. 1d

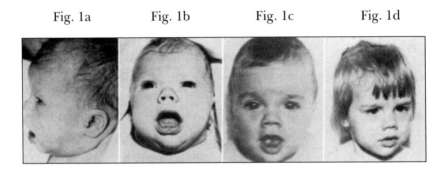

Fig. 1e   Fig. 1f

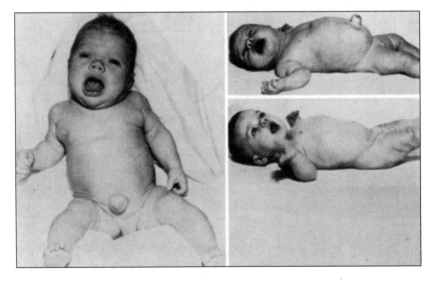

Fig. 1g

Source: Lisser, H., and Escamilla, R. *Atlas of Clinical Endocrinology*, C. V. Mosby Company, 1957. Reprinted with permission.

Figures 1a and 1b show the deep-set nose (saddle nose), puffy lips, and thick protruding tongue. The child weighed over nine pounds at birth. At nine months of age, she was unable to sit up or hold her head erect. The posterior fontanel remained open. No teeth had erupted. Her rectal temperature was 96.4 °F (35.8 °C). BMR was minus 45%. Her cholesterol dropped from 210 mg% to 168 mg% after 11 days of thyroid therapy.

Figure 1c shows the child after 5.5 months of treatment with desiccated thyroid (0.3 grains increased to 0.75 grains). Note the loss of puffiness and the more prominent bridge of her nose.

Figure 1d is taken after 21 months of treatment (age 2 years 7 months). Her mouth is almost closed. The lips are no longer puffy, and the tongue is no longer visible. Sixteen teeth are now present, as is evidence of increased scalp hair growth. Her height is now 32 inches (a growth of 10 inches in 21 months).

Figure 1e shows her appearance in the sitting position before treatment. Note the narrow eye slits, pug nose, wide-open mouth, large tongue, protuberant abdomen, and umbilical hernia (all are features of hypothyroidism).

Figure 1f shows the child in the lying position before treatment. She had dry, coarse, cold skin.

Figure 1g shows the disappearance of the umbilical hernia and flattening of the stomach after 5.5 months of desiccated thyroid therapy. She had grown 4.5 inches.

Skin problems are abundant. Dry skin (especially on the elbows and knees), eczema, psoriasis, or infections involving the skin or scalp are clues. The skin may be pale and the extremities are usually cool to the touch. The palms and soles of the feet are occasionally yellowed.

Respiration may be noisy due to swollen nasal passages. Babies may breathe entirely through their mouths and appear to have a constant cold.

Eyesight and hearing problems are common. Cataracts were formerly the province of the aged. They, too, may be associated with hypothyroidism and often occur in premature babies. Dr. Zondek stated, "Very close associations exist between cretinism and deaf-mutism, since a high incidence of goitre coincides regionally with that of deaf-mutism." Abnormalities in the shape of the outer ear (pinna) are common.[8,35]

Not infrequently a child's **jaw or teeth are unable to develop normally**. The crowding together of teeth has been associated by anthropologists with the modernization of civilization. I have also seen the opposite, large gaps between the teeth in a few of my patients. Both should now be associated with hypothyroidism. **Irritated gums, enlarged gums, gums projecting between the teeth, multiple cavities, and delayed dental development are red flags.** Occasionally, problems with delayed dental development or cavities may be the first sign of hypothyroidism in an otherwise healthy child. The teeth and jaw begin normal development after dessicated thyroid is administered.

Constipation or other problems with the digestive tract are among the most common symptoms. In his 1914 lecture, Dr. Hertoghe mentioned the slowness of digestion as well as scant secretions in the intestines of affected children. He stated, "These may lead to development of false membranes and then grow into bands causing kinks and other consequences." In the same lecture, he described another physical feature often present in hypothyroid infants, including cretins. **A protuberant abdomen**, so common today, was his observation.

As a child develops, **bed-wetting, poor coordination, and swallowing problems may develop. Morning fatigue, difficulty awakening, or sleepwalking are possible.**

A listing of symptoms with regard to hypothyroidism in infants is found on the next page. This list is from a modern medical textbook and is limited but revealing.

Table 8.1 **The Thyroid: Infant Hypothyroidism Symptoms**

Early Neonatal Appearance
  Edema [swelling]
  Gestation > 42 wk.
  Birth weight > 4 kg [8.8 lbs.]
  Poor feeding
  Hypothermia [low temperature]
  Abdominal distention
  Large posterior fontanel

Onset during the First Month of Age
  Peripheral cyanosis and mottling [blotchy, cold arms
    and legs]
  Respiratory distress
  Failure to gain weight and poor sucking ability
  Decreased stool frequency
  Decreased activity and lethargy

Onset during the First Three Months of Age
  Umbilical hernia
  Constipation
  Dry and sallow [yellowed] skin
  Macroglossia [large tongue]
  Generalized myxedema [non-pitting swelling, refer to
    Chapter 1]
  Hoarse cry

Onset during Childhood
  Growth retardation with delayed skeletal maturation
  Delayed dental development and tooth eruption
  Constipation
  Generalized myxedema
  Precocious sexual development
  Muscle dysfunction and abnormal muscle enlargement

Source: Braverman, Lewis, E., Utiger, and Robert, D. *Warner & Ingbar's The Thyroid: A Fundamental and Clinical Text.* 8th ed. Philadelphia: Lippincott Williams & Wilkins, 2000. Reprinted with permission.

A listing of symptoms from another text on congenital (inherited) hypothyroidism follows:

Table 8.2   **The Thyroid and Its Diseases**
Signs and Symptoms of Congenital Hypothyroidism in Infants

Symptoms	Number of Infants	Translation by Dr. Starr
Constipation	9/22	
Lethargy	7/22	
Prolonged jaundice	6/21	
Poor feeding	5/22	
Temperature <36 °C	1/12	<96.8 °F
Large anterior fontanel	4/18	
Large posterior fontanel	2/17	
Macroglossia	4/21	Large tongue
Goiter	0/21	Thyroid growth in front of neck
Umbilical hernia	6/21	Belly button outpouching
Hypotonia	7/21	Decreased tone or laxity of muscles
Slow relaxation of deep tendon reflexes	3/21	Delayed relaxation of reflexes (especially ankle reflexes)

Source: DeGroot, L. J., Larsen, P. R., and Hennemann, G. *The Thyroid and Its Diseases*. Sixth Edition; New York: Churchill Livingstone Inc., 1996, page 559. Reprinted with permission.

The fact that the recent literature regarding hypothyroidism now considers a temperature above 96.8 °F (36 °C) instead of 97.8 °F to be normal is of special interest. It is a classic demonstration of how the hypothyroid state has now been accepted as normal.

All parents should read Dr. Barnes' book on hypothyroidism for their children's sake, if not their own. The 36 °C (96.8 °F) listed in Table 8.2 from the modern textbook is erroneous. As previously stated, rectal temperatures are 0.8 to 1.0 °F higher than axillary temperature, i.e., 98.6 °F is the absolute minimum for a normal rectal test with a thermometer. Refer to the section on basal temperature for details.

The telltale symptoms of hypothyroidism may not be apparent for decades. Unfortunately, as the epidemic worsens, the symptoms are occurring in younger age groups and are more severe.

Adolescents

Puberty, pregnancy, and menopause place increased demands upon thyroid hormone functions. A child may seem to be relatively well until puberty when a number of behavioral and physical problems will suddenly appear.

Again, disturbances of growth, problems involving sexual development, and mental disturbances are paramount features of hypothyroidism.

Growth Disturbances

Laxity of the ligaments that help support our bones as well as muscular imbalances result from hypothyroidism. The end result may be hyper-flexibility, scoliosis, stooped posture, knock-kneed legs, chronic pain and a tendency to sprain or strain which may frequently linger. The kneecaps may spontaneously dislocate. I have seen two such patients, both with undiagnosed Type 2 hypothyroidism. The senior Dr. Hertoghe stated, "The ligaments at the internal aspect of the knee-joints are those most frequently affected, with the result that a certain amount of knock-knee becomes apparent." The same article featured pictures of a patient with both kneecaps dislocated.[2]

"Adolescent idiopathic scoliosis" occurs in 2% to 3% of our children by age 16. It is the most common form of scoliosis, an abnormal curvature of the spine. Idiopathic means doctors and scientists do not know the cause of an illness.

Scoliosis is two to three times more common among adolescent girls than among adolescent boys. The onset of the illness is usually during puberty. My assumption is that the vast majority of those affected suffer many other symptoms of hypothyroidism and run low basal temperatures. My brother as well as several of my patients suffering scoliosis fit this profile.

Hypothyroidism may cause growth plates at the ends of our long bones to close prematurely or remain open longer than normal. This may result in very short or very tall stature depending upon genetic factors and the severity of an individual's hypothyroidism. Despite having a father of almost six feet and a mother five feet five inches, my growth stopped before age 15 at five feet seven inches. I'm the shortest male on both sides of large families. My parents were concerned enough to take me to several doctors in an attempt to find an explanation. The answer given was "natural variation". An endocrinologist advised against the possible use of growth hormone due to possible side effects. The year was 1967. Unfortunately, a blood test was my only examination for hypothyroidism.

One of my adolescent patients was short for her age, overweight, had frequent upper respiratory infections, and felt cold and tired for as long as she could recall. After two years of treatment with desiccated thyroid, she had grown over four inches, lost nine pounds, was no longer cold or tired, and had only missed one or two days of school due to illness.

Growth hormone is now widely used to treat children with short stature. Without exception, the children I have seen who were treated with growth hormone have been hypothyroid. Thyroid hormones would have allowed normal growth to proceed in addition to resolution of all the other manifestations of the illness they continued to suffer.

Sexual Development

Dr. Zondek mentioned general contraction of the pelvis as another prominent physical feature. Many women have small pelvic bones and narrow hips. This condition often portends problems with childbirth.

As stated, hypothyroidism may cause premature or delayed puberty. The majority of normal and hypothyroid females begin their cycles at ages 12 or 13. However, a growing number of those with hypothyroidism start their cycle years earlier or begin their periods at age 15 or later. Premature or delayed puberty in males is also becoming more common.

Problems associated with the menstrual cycle are now commonplace. The majority of the teenagers whom I have seen suffer problems such as PMS, severe cramping, and irregular or heavy cycles. Severe hypothyroidism may cause the menses to cease. Dr. Barnes devoted a whole chapter in his book to menstrual disorders and problems with fertility. He noted his patients with menstrual problems usually suffered many other telltale symptoms of hypothyroidism. Mine do so as well.

A large majority of menstrual problems resolve after treatment with desiccated thyroid (iodine replacement is also crucial). Much more detail is provided in the following section about adult hypothyroidism entitled "Menstrual Disorders and Fertility".

The following pictures are illustrative of a severely affected 14 year-old hypothyroid girl.

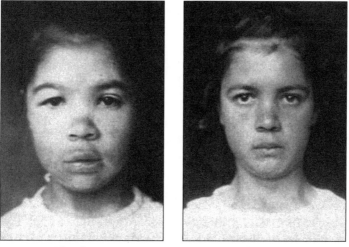

Fig. 2a   Fig. 2b

Source: Lisser, H., and Escamilla, R. *Atlas of Clinical Endocrinology*, C. V. Mosby Company, 1957. Reprinted with permission.

Figure 2a shows the 14 year-old before treatment. Note the saddle nose, puffiness around the eyes, thickened lips, and straight coarse hair. She suffered very heavy menstrual flow lasting seven or eight days, occurring every three months since age 12. She was severely constipated, had mild anemia, and was slightly overweight despite a poor appetite.

Figure 2b shows her appearance after six months of thyroid therapy. Note the elevated bridge of the nose, brighter eyes, thinner lips, and glossy, curly hair. The constipation resolved and her appetite improved. There was no mention of changes in menstrual cycle by the authors.

The sex organs may develop normally but are often smaller than normal. Dr. Zondek stated, "The development of the genital system is disturbed in most cases. Both the internal and external genital organs are hypoplastic (underdeveloped), and so are the mammae (breasts). In exceptional cases, however, I have seen genital development exceeding the normal limits."[8] Dr. Eugene Hertoghe cited retroflexion of the uterus (the top is bent backwards) as a developmental problem also associated with hypothyroidism.[32] Several of my patients suffered retroflexion and other developmental defects of the uterus.

Mentation

Hypothyroidism may not cause any mental disturbance. The mental changes may be mild or only become evident at a much later age. However, statistics show mental problems are beginning earlier and increasing in severity. Suicide is now the third leading cause of death among 10 to 24 year-old Americans.

There is a laundry list of mental problems linked to hypothyroidism. Many of these mental infirmities are no longer linked to hypothyroidism in the newer literature. Nervousness and irritability are common as are apathy and listlessness. Problems with memory or problems performing tasks, which were done previously without effort, are additional signs. Our National Institute of Mental Health estimates that 8% of adolescents have symptoms of depression. Many other serious conditions are possible. Delusions, hallucinations (both auditory and visual), and frank insanity are only a sample.

Dr. Zondek stated, "In spite of pronounced signs of the disease many patients retain their memory, judgment, and other mental faculties intact. But with progress of the disease these, too, are impaired. Not uncommonly the emotions become unbalanced, occasionally genuine psychosis develops. The patients may then become depressed or, more rarely, maniacal and have outbreaks of passion, rage, and even fury. Various forms of distressing obsessions have been recorded."[8] More discussion about mental affectations is in the next section: Adult Hypothyroidism.

Dr. Barnes, as well as other researchers, documented the hypothyroids' propensity toward alcohol and substance abuse. Early researchers noted alcoholic beverages diminished hypothyroid symptoms. Dr. Barnes stated that he never treated an alcoholic patient who was not hypothyroid.[55]

Alcoholic drinks tend to induce low blood sugar (glucose) in normal individuals. Hypothyroid individuals are usually even more sensitive to the deleterious effects of alcohol.

Dr. Barnes felt that much of the carnage on our nation's highways, as well as a good deal of criminal behavior, was due in part to our growing hypothyroid population's tendency toward hypoglycemia (low blood sugar). Hypoglycemia is greatly exacerbated by alcohol. The brain is dependent upon a constant supply of glucose, a form of sugar. Aberrant behavior, hallucinations, and passing out are just a few of the symptoms that may result from a shortage of glucose to the brain. Dr. Barnes speaks at length about the relationship between alcohol, hypothyroidism, and hypoglycemia in his book, *Hope for Hypoglycemia*. He presented a mountain of evidence that hypoglycemia is one of the many possible symptoms of hypothyroidism. Hypoglycemia resolved after proper treatment with thyroid hormones and no new cases developed in any patients who were already being treated for their hypothyroidism.[55]

Tobacco use may also be associated with hypothyroidism. Nicotine momentarily helps the chronic fatigue associated with hypothyroidism. Dr. Barnes found that his patients were much better able to stop smoking when their hypothyroidism and "damnable fatigue" resolved. I was able to stop my smoking habit of 30 years after treatment with desiccated thyroid.

Adult Hypothyroidism

The symptoms of adult hypothyroidism may be applicable to adolescents or children and the reverse may be true. Untreated hypothyroidism worsens with age. Mild symptoms gradually worsen with the passing of time. Many of my patients stated they had been cold, constipated, or suffered dry skin for as long as they could remember.

Occasionally, there may be a sudden change for the worse such as in autoimmune thyroiditis, also known as Hashimoto's Disease. For some "unknown reason," the body decides to destroy its own thyroid gland. This entity is thought to cause the majority of the adult Type 1 hypothyroidism as recognized by mainstream medicine. Hashimoto's disease also tends to run in families. The immune system and the endocrine glands are adversely affected by Type 2 hypothyroidism. The patients I treated who suffered autoimmune thyroiditis have histories consistent with Type 2 hypothyroidism.

I wrote the first draft of this book in Columbia, Missouri. My office windows overlooked the University of Missouri campus. The "characteristic physiognomy" (appearance) of hypothyroidism was common among the thousands of students who passed by my window. Thirty years prior, I had begun college there. The increase in students' height and obesity in the intervening period was quite striking. Numerous other physical changes associated with hypothyroidism such as contraction of the pelvis (narrow hips) in women were also apparent.

Symptoms frequently are exacerbated by cold weather. Cold places an increased demand upon thyroid function, due to the additional energy required to heat our bodies. Remember that the thyroid hormones are responsible for our energy production.

Many times I witnessed four prime examples of the hypothyroid state: seasonal depression (wintertime); asthma which is much worse in cold weather; dry itchy skin (often termed winter itch); and more frequent infections such as colds, sinus infections, and pneumonia. No wonder our population has gravitated toward warmer climates.

Dr. Sonkin stated in a journal article that the most common complaints associated with a possible diagnosis of hypothyroidism were chronic pain, depression, fatigue, loss of energy, cold intolerance, constipation, and dry puffy skin (myxedema).[56]

After two years of study and treatment in New York, I began private practice in 1996. Initially, I would ask new patients if they suffered these symptoms. If they responded negatively, I would look no further. Gradually, it became apparent that many patients were unaware of their hypothyroid symptoms. The symptoms had been present for years, and patients assumed they were normal constituents of aging, or that was just the way they were. A much more detailed questionnaire and physical exam became necessary. Dr. Kraus had cautioned me to be aware of the fact that a person might only exhibit one symptom of hypothyroidism and yet require treatment.

My hands are usually no longer cold, which makes it possible for me to touch a patient's hands, feet, extremities, or torso and easily tell if they are abnormally cool. I pinch the skin on the lateral upper arm and the front of the thighs looking for abnormal thickness. In more advanced cases, it may be difficult to lift the skin in order to pinch at all. The tissues are adherent or stuck to the underlying structures because of the infiltration of the glue-like substance, mucin. The majority of my new patients' temperatures are below 97.8 °F when taken in my office. Their basal temperatures are usually even lower.

All the following symptoms in this chapter have a long list of possible causes. However, if you have a low basal temperature and symptoms of hypothyroidism; or a low temperature and family history of thyroid related problems, I believe a trial of thyroid hormones is indicated.

The Face

The appearance of one's face is often markedly affected. Swelling above the eyes and less often, below the eyes may occur. The eyelids, upper and lower, may be thickened or take on an oblique direction. In some cases, individuals must tilt their heads back in order to keep the eyes open. The face appears puffy due in large part to the deposition of myxedema along the jaw line. The lips may be pale or swollen and the nostrils broadened. In Caucasians, the skin of the face is often pale. However, a pink flush may be present over the cheeks, which ends at the lower margins of the eyes. The mobility of the features, particularly of the mouth may be limited. The ends of the lips may turn downward as if pouting. The ears may be swollen and stand out. The hair gradually loses its natural gloss, becomes brittle, and progressively thins, almost to the point of baldness. Many variations of these changes in milder forms are common. Once one becomes familiar with the characteristic appearance of hypothyroidism, it should be as obvious as the myxedema on your face. As previously stated, a large percentage of affected patients do not exhibit external puffiness.[2,3,8,48]

The following pictures are from the senior Dr. Hertoghe's 1915 medical journal article. They illustrate the characteristic appearance of hypothyroidism "upon first glance". The resolution of puffiness or myxedema is quite striking.[2]

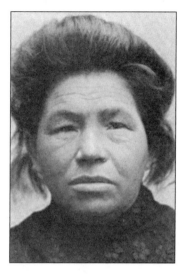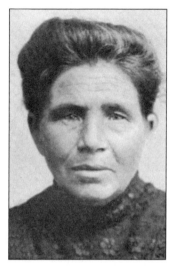

Before treatment   After treatment

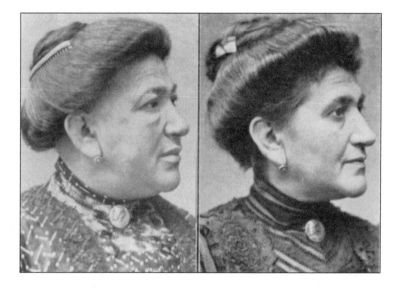

Before treatment   After treatment

Source: Hertoghe, E. *The Practitioner*, Jan 1915, Vol XCIV, No 1, 26-93

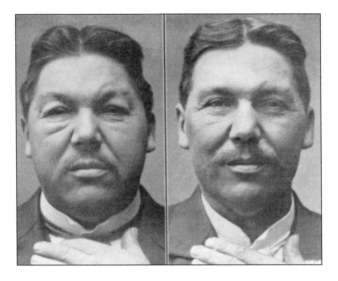

Before treatment   After treatment

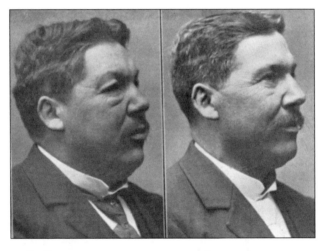

Before treatment   After treatment

Source: Hertoghe, E. *The Practitioner*, Jan 1915, Vol XCIV, No 1, 26-93.

The next case from the atlas of Drs. Lisser and Escamilla illustrates the amazing results that may be attained from desiccated thyroid treatment.[48]

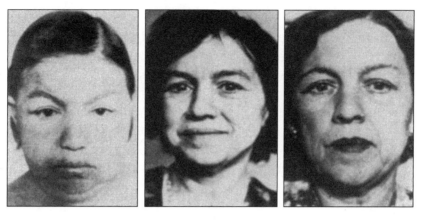

Fig. 3a   Fig. 3b   Fig. 3c

Source: Lisser, H., and Escamilla, R. Atlas of Clinical Endocrinology, C. V. Mosby Company, 1957. Reprinted with permission.

Figure 3a shows an unmarried woman, age 34. Her only complaint was stiffness and weakness in her knees when climbing stairs. She exhibited the puffy face, coarse, straight hair, short neck, a deep and leathery voice, an umbilical hernia, and had no pubic or axillary (armpits) hair. Her menses began at age 16 and were irregular. She felt cold. Her mental age was 12 years, and her bone age (on X-rays) was 10 years. She had a BMR of minus 39%, a heart rate of 60, and she had anemia.

Figure 3b shows the woman after nine months of desiccated thyroid treatment (2 grains daily). The patient's expression became alert and animated, her puffiness was gone, pubic hair had appeared, the anemia resolved, and she married nine months later.

Figure 3c shows the woman at age 46, 12 years after beginning treatment. Her BMR was now plus 1%.

The Skin

Hypothyroidism decreases circulation. Our bodies shunt blood away from the skin and toward the brain and vital internal organs as circulation is diminished. In advanced cases of hypothyroidism, the skin may receive only 20% of its normal blood supply.[4]

Increased susceptibility to skin infection is a hallmark of hypothyroidism. Boils and acne were common in my patients and their families.

With thyroid treatment, Dr. Barnes cured 90% of his patients who suffered all degrees of acne. He and the doctors Hertoghe associated many other skin disorders such as eczema, psoriasis, impetigo, and cellulitis (subcutaneous tissue infections) with the disease. Many of my patients had acne as teens. Dr. Barnes devoted an entire chapter to skin problems. As Dr. Hertoghe stated, "The whole skin is thickened, infiltrated, cold, and easily attacked by such affectations as eczema, psoriasis, and alopecia [hair loss]."[32]

Dr. Barnes treated 12 patients for psoriasis. Eight showed marked improvement or cleared completely. The majority of these skin problems are also familial (tend to be inherited).

Several of my patients stated that dermatologists had given up on the treatment of their acne, eczema, or psoriatic conditions. Proper thyroid treatment cleared or significantly improved the majority of their skin problems. As the epidemic worsens, these conditions will become more common.

The face is usually the first place where puffiness or myxedema begins, most often above or below the eyes. I can't help but notice this telltale appearance in friends, family, television stars, professional athletes, doctors, etc.

When shown how thick her skin was, a patient commented, "I wondered why my dermatologist had such a problem stitching it together after removing a benign growth."

A tendency to develop allergies is also associated with hypothyroidism. A patient of mine was tested for allergies at a large environmental medical center. The upper-lateral arm is used to inject allergy extracts under the skin. The woman, doing the testing, commented that my patient's skin was strange, because it was thin and "rolled around". My patient had been on desiccated thyroid for years. The myxedema present in the other patients was lacking in my patient's skin.

As the disease progresses, "parchment-like" fine wrinkles appear, one of the many characteristics of premature aging caused by hypothyroidism. The wrinkles are most evident on the face and hands.

Several patients of mine asked why they had a bulge or puffiness above their collarbones on the front of their necks. I didn't have an answer initially. However, my studies uncovered the fact that hypothyroidism frequently causes "fat pads" above the collarbones (clavicles).

Severely affected patients may take on a yellowish or amber tint to their skin. This is due to the inability to convert beta-carotene into vitamin A by the liver. The liver becomes congested and more dysfunctional as the severity of hypothyroidism increases.

The absence of, or diminished, perspiration was first described in the 1888 report and remains a common feature of hypothyroidism. Excessive perspiration is less frequent. The effects of the disease are often paradoxical even among siblings.

Patients learn to live with their dry skin and are often well lubricated with lotion when they present themselves at my office. Their hands, feet, and lower legs, just above the ankles, are the first places I look for dry skin. Elbows and knees are frequently affected. Check the feel of the skin on your elbow with the arm bent. Normally, the skin feels the same as the skin on the rest of the arm.

Vitiligo, "a usually progressive, chronic pigmentation anomaly of the skin, manifested by depigmented white patches," is another possible symptom. Mine was not progressive.

Skin cancers are now epidemic, and their incidence continues to rise. Almost without exception, my patients who were previously diagnosed with skin cancer had subnormal temperatures as well as other symptomatology of hypothyroidism. The impairment of our immune system from hypothyroidism, environmental toxins, and decreased circulation (up to 80%) to the skin must surely contribute mightily.

Melanomas are by far the deadliest form of skin cancer. Ten years ago, the occurrence rate was one in 250. Today, the rate is one in 76 and predicted to increase to 1 in 50. The U.S. Center for Disease Control estimates the increased frequency of melanoma is 3% per year. People who have a large number of moles are at increased risk. In the original 1888 report, abundant moles and warty growths on the skin were noted physical findings associated with hypothyroidism. From Dr. Ord's 1901 chapter entitled Myxoedema, "Moles are often developed, especially on the trunk." Moles tend to be hereditary affectations.[7]

The persistent dogma continues to blame sunburns, especially in childhood, for the explosion of melanomas. However, unlike most skin cancers, melanomas often occur in areas that receive little sun such as the palms, soles of the feet, toes, vulva, vagina, esophagus, anus, or inside the mouth. Many of my patients or their family members have suffered this cancer. Although sunburns may promote melanoma, in my opinion the principal underlying problem appears to be Type 2 hypothyroidism and iodine deficiencies.

The Hair

Premature baldness and diffuse hair loss are symptoms. A recent statistic stated that 40% of American women are suffering significant hair loss by the age of 40. More photographs from Dr. Hertoghe's 1915 journal article show the powerful effect thyroid hormones have on hair and physical features when properly administered.

The frontal views and profiles of two patients, before treatment and following treatment, are on the next page. Note the puffiness (myxedema) in their faces and hands resolves.

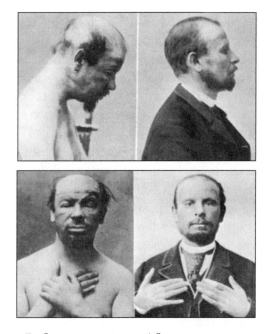

Before treatment   After treatment

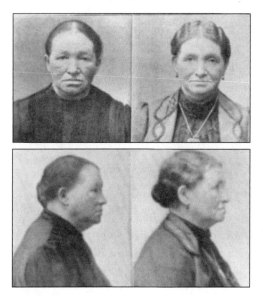

Before treatment   After treatment

Source: Hertoghe, E. *The Practitioner*, Jan 1915, Vol XCIV, No 1, 26-93.

Fine, thin, straight, dry hair often results from mild hypothyroidism. Coarse hair may be a manifestation of more severe cases. Notice the curly, thicker hair in the woman after treatment. In advanced hypothyroidism, the person loses hair from the front of their head as well as the back (the nape of the neck). Individuals may end up with a strip of hair across the middle of their heads.

One former patient comes to mind who suffered severe hair loss. The patient was a friendly 67 year-old farmer's wife who typifies the reason for my writing this book. She entered my office complaining of right arm and hand pain. Questioning revealed increasing cold intolerance, dry skin, thinning hair, fatigue, high blood pressure, migraine headaches, hypoglycemia, prior lower back surgery, prior TIA (a transient stroke), skin cancer, iron deficiency anemia, vitamin B12 deficiency, as well as a family history of diabetes and heart disease. Physical findings included diffuse hair loss, extremely dry hair and skin with mild myxedema (puffiness), cold hands and feet, claw toes, and diffuse muscle tenderness. She also had a son who suffered from chronic fatigue syndrome (CFS). Her basal temperature was barely 96 °F degrees when she checked it.

In medical textbooks, iron deficiency anemia and B12 deficiency are associated with hypothyroidism. She received injections of iron and B12 for years, in addition to suffering many of the hallmarks representing hypothyroidism. And yet, because of normal blood tests, the patient was never offered treatment for hypothyroidism. Within six months of treatment, the patient improved remarkably.

Another important physical finding closely associated with hypothyroidism is the thinning or loss of the outside third of the eyebrows. In some patients the eyebrows are absent. Modern medical textbooks refer to the loss of the outer eyebrow as "Queen Anne's sign". However, this sign was first noted by Dr. Eugene Hertoghe and was mentioned in his 1914 lecture and 1915 journal article. Endocrinologists in the know refer to this sign as the "Sign of Hertoghe".[2,32]

Typical facial appearance of hypothyroidism including loss of eye brows is shown in the following patients.

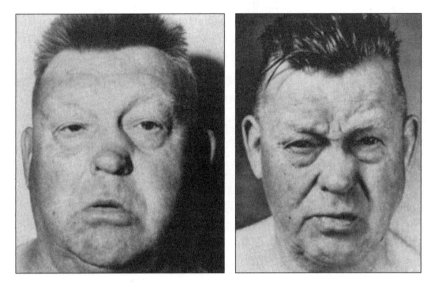

Fig. 4a
Before treatment

Fig. 4b
After treatment

Source: Lisser, H., and Escamilla, R. *Atlas of Clinical Endocrinology*, C. V. Mosby Company, 1957. Reprinted with permission.

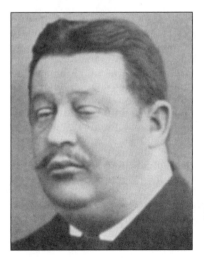

Myxedema in a 49 year-old man.

Source: Zondek, H. 1944. *Diseases of the Endocrine Glands*, 4th ed. Baltimore: The Williams and Wilkins Company. Reprinted with permission.

Figure 4a shows a 56 year-old hypothyroid man with scant eyebrows, puffiness (myxedema) around the eyes and face, and down-turned corners of the mouth.

Figure 4b shows the patient after five months of treatment with 2 grains of desiccated thyroid. Note the resolution of myxedema. The scalp hair and eyebrows have grown, although the lateral eyebrows have not yet filled in.

Many patients gradually lose the hair from their lower legs, arms, and armpits in varying degrees. For years, I had believed the missing hair on the back of my calves must have been the result of constant rubbing from my pants. The hair has returned with proper thyroid replacement and without changing my wardrobe.

As previously mentioned, dry, coarse, brittle hair often develops. However, a number of hypothyroid patients had an abundance of healthy hair, especially the younger ones.

The Nails

The condition of my patients' nails is usually affected in one way or another. The big toenail often is affected first. Several of my patients had their big toenails removed due to chronic ingrown toenails and fungal infections. I suffered ingrown toenails during my younger years.

Healthy nails are translucent, clear, shiny, firm, and smooth. The nail beds are pink when blood circulation is up to snuff. Hypothyroidism gradually leaves the nails pale or yellowish, brittle, ridged, striated, and thickened. They peel or break easily. The nails may be soft due to associated iron deficiency.

The Eyes

Healthy eyes are bright, clear, and shiny. Red, irritated, dry eyes are suspect. Visual disturbances and night vision problems are frequent. Again, hypothyroid patients are unable to convert beta-carotene into vitamin A, which is necessary for vision especially at night.

Glaucoma and cataracts may result. Blepharitis, conjunctivitis, and other infections involving the eyes become more common with age as do other symptoms of hypothyroidism.

From Dr. Hertoghe's 1914 lecture: "The eyelashes are also shed, leaving the eyelids unprotected against the erosive action of the tears. This blepharitis of thyroid origin is sometimes seen in old persons."[32]

Neurological problems such as macular degeneration, spasm of the eyelids (blepharospasm), or drooping of the eyelid are much more likely to occur. Every patient that I have seen with these conditions suffered hypothyroidism, in my opinion.

The eyelids often become swollen. People may struggle to hold their eyes open or tilt their head backward in order to see. Their eyelids may acquire an oblique direction as described by Dr. Ord, "such as seen in Mongolian tribes." The following pictures are from Dr. Ord's treatise on myxedema published in 1901.[7]

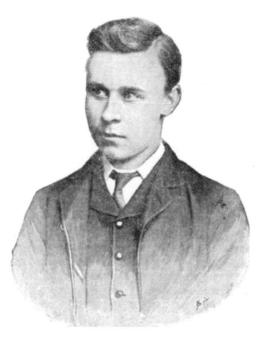

Before onset of hypothyroidism

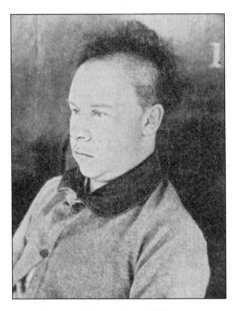

Severe hypothyroidism

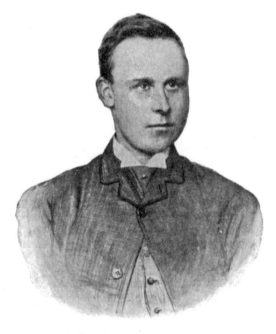

Following treatment

The Ears and Hearing

Type 2 hypothyroidism can result in the ears being located lower than normal on our head. Occasionally, they almost appear to be originating from the upper neck. The following pictures of an adult cretin taken from Dr. Zondek's text illustrates their lower than normal position.[8]

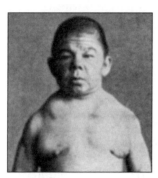
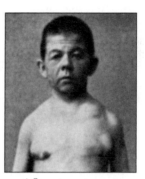

Before treatment   After treatment

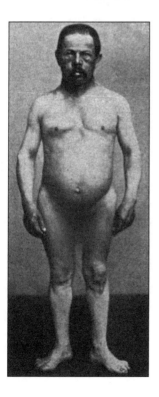
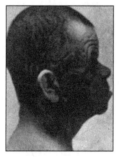
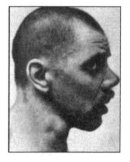

Above: Side profile of two cretins.

Source: Lisser, H., and Escamilla, R. *Atlas of Clinical Endocrinology*, C. V. Mosby Company, 1957. Reprinted with permission.

Left: Adult cretin. Note flat feet, knock-knee, and short legs.

Source: Zondek, H. 1944. *Diseases of the Endocrine Glands*, 4th ed. Baltimore: The Williams and Wilkins Company. Reprinted with permission.

In advanced cases, the ears may be swollen and stand out with marked prominence. The ear canal may be dry, scaly, and may itch. Excess formation of earwax is often reduced to normal levels after treatment of hypothyroidism. The earwax (cerumen) problem I used to suffer from required a nurse to periodically flush it out. My ear syringe has not been used in many years, as my ears now produce only small, normal amounts of cerumen.

Recurrent infections may begin at an early age or may begin much later. Ear infections may contribute to hearing loss. Deafness or other hearing deficits may be attributable to low thyroid function. I used a combination of white vinegar and isopropyl alcohol after showers and swimming to avoid the recurrent ear infections that had formerly plagued me. I have not had an ear infection since beginning desiccated thyroid treatment.

Tinnitus (ringing in the ears) is another common and prominently listed symptom of hypothyroidism. In my limited experience with this symptom, the more long-standing the problem, the less likely it is to resolve. However, the progression of this problem may be significantly delayed or halted.

The Teeth, Gums, and TMJ Syndrome

Diminished immunity against infection, impaired ability to repair damaged tissues, poor circulation, and other factors associated with hypothyroidism all contribute to poor oral health. Many of my patients reported horror stories regarding their dentition. Their teeth literally rotted one by one, occasionally in rapid succession. The vast majority of these adults all suffered the usual constellation of hypothyroid symptoms.

The propensity for cavities and gum disease was established by The Committee of the Clinical Society of London's Report in 1888. "Their teeth usually suffer in their nutrition, and break off, fall, or become carious [decayed]. The gums are often swollen, spongy and bleeding, and occasionally receding."[1] These symptoms of periodontal disease have been linked to heart attacks (another innocent bystander convicted by circumstantial evidence).

Overdeveloped gums, which project downward between the teeth, are telltale signs. These "polypoid projections" of the gums are cited in the early literature. I notice increasingly enlarged gums, occasionally to the point where the teeth barely emerge, in the younger generations.[1,2,32]

Temporomandibular Joint Dysfunction (TMJ), muscle pain, and their relation to hypothyroidism were addressed by Dr. Sonkin in a book written by a famous dentist at NYU, Harold Gelb, D.M.D. Dr. Kraus also contributed a chapter and collaborated with these two pioneers. This team of a muscle pain specialist (Kraus), endocrinologist (Sonkin), dentist (Gelb), and the physical and psychological therapists with whom they worked, probably comprised the most talented TMJ treatment group in medical history.[6]

Dr. Sonkin believed muscular dysfunction and tension resulting from hypothyroidism were major underlying factors in the development of TMJ syndrome. The basis for this belief was due to the increased incidence of jaw muscle spasms, muscular tension and pain that are often associated with hypothyroidism. I managed to crack both of my lower back molars before proper thyroid treatment resolved the problem. Twenty-five percent of my pain patients complained of teeth clenching and TMJ pain. However, TMJ was rarely their primary complaint.

I met with a local dentist who specialized in the treatment of TMJ not long after opening my practice. Patients frequently require special dental devices to help protect, and often realign, their teeth. I hoped to discuss a mutually satisfactory working arrangement in order to invoke both of our specialties to aid remediation of our patients' TMJ syndromes. The dentist's response to my query was, "The underlying cause of TMJ is now well established. I published several papers on the subject [which he presented to me]. A high-resolution, thin slice MRI has proven that almost all women have demonstrable degenerative changes [arthritic] in both of their temporomandibular joints by the age of 30." He continued, "Dentists have not yet figured out why many of these women suffer pain in only one joint, which frequently shows less arthritis than the other." Gathering my papers, I thanked him for his time. Obviously, Dr. Sonkin's research relating hormone deficiencies to muscle involvement had once again fallen on deaf ears. Doesn't the fact that women with TMJ often suffer more pain in the less arthritic joint point toward muscular involvement? The high prevalence of arthritic changes in women's temporomandibular joints by age 30 may be another indication of the epidemic of Type 2 hypothyroidism (refer to section on arthritis for details).

TMJ and teeth clenching often gradually resolve following treatment with desiccated thyroid. The addition of estrogen for postmenopausal women may be necessary for relief. Additional treatments such as physical therapy, trigger point injections, prolotherapy (injections into ligaments), and supportive dental care also help this difficult problem.

Normal development and function of the jaw, teeth, and muscles are promoted by proper treatment of hypothyroidism in the young.

The Speech, Tongue, and Swallowing

Hoarseness is a frequent symptom. The vocal cords become swollen and infiltrated with mucin. At age 41, my hoarseness became very bothersome until treatment with thyroid hormones resolved the problem. Thoughts of untreated hypothyroidism cross my mind when I watch television and hear someone with a hoarse voice, particularly when there is puffiness around the face or eyes. Dr. Barnes cited a patient whose vocal cord was biopsied in an attempt to find a cause for her hoarseness. He stated, "The diagnosis was written all over her face."[10]

Dr. Ord described the effects of severe hypothyroidism as, "The speech is altered in so uniform a way that a diagnosis may almost be made when a patient, unseen, is heard talking. The words come very slowly and deliberately, the voice is monotonous and of a leathery timbre, no doubt much determined by the swelling of the throat, and is evidently produced with considerable effort owing to the swelling of the lips. This can be recognized if the patient is watched as he speaks, the words seeming to be squeezed out of the lips with much difficulty. As already mentioned, there is probably a nervous as well as a mechanical cause for the change in speech."[7]

Speech problems abound. Difficulties with pronunciation or pattern such as slow, halting speech are often a result of hypothyroidism. High pitched or nasal voices may have been much different had thyroid hormones been given during the maturation process.

The tongue may be abnormally large. The side of your tongue may be scalloped due to pressure from the teeth, small jaw, and myxedema. In severe cases, the swollen tongue tends to fall backward and obstruct breathing.

Problems swallowing are not infrequent. A combination of swelling of the esophagus and impaired function of the associated nerves may be a minor bother or may wreak havoc. I successfully treated a 10 year-old for this problem. His recurrent infections and fatigue also resolved. More commonly, it is the aged who are most affected. My mother's progressive problem swallowing pills slowly resolved after beginning desiccated thyroid hormones.

Mental and Neurological Symptoms

A network of supporting structures, including blood vessels and nutrient supplying cells, surround our nerves. These structures, which provide oxygen and essential nutrients, become progressively infiltrated with mucin. The function and health of the nerves suffer. Autopsy studies across Western Civilization from the late nineteenth century and early twentieth century, 70,000 Graz autopsies reviewed by Dr. Barnes, and countless other autopsies on man and other mammals are all unequivocal concerning this characteristic of hypothyroidism.

A very gradual decline in a person's energy, often followed by listlessness may be the first indication of a problem. Declines in the ability to concentrate as well as fatigue are also frequent scenarios. Memory loss was first documented in the report of 1888. The report stated, "Memory is usually impaired from an early period of the disease, especially in respect of recent events."[1]

One of the first signs of dementia is short-term memory loss. Alzheimer's disease, dementia, as well as mental illnesses frequently run in families, as does hypothyroidism. The problem has become magnified due to the severity of the hypothyroidism epidemic and modern medicine's ability to keep patients alive. Half of Americans 85 years or older are suffering from Alzheimer's, which is tragically beginning to strike at younger and younger ages.

For example, my father's mental status was declining in his early 80s. Proper treatment of his hypothyroidism and other hormone deficiencies (DHEA and testosterone) reversed his mental decline and restored his sense of humor. My mother thanked me many times for giving her husband back to her. Restoring quality of life is gratifying even if one's life expectancy is limited.

Tension and irritability are closely associated with the hypothyroid state. Drs. Barnes and Sonkin blamed nervous tension for the erroneously high basal metabolism tests, nervousness, tremor, and other seemingly paradoxical symptoms found in many hypothyroid patients. They believed this tension was due to overcompensation by the adrenal glands in an effort to increase the body's metabolism.

Depression was present in over half of my pain patients. Most had already tried multiple antidepressants with limited success. Patients, friends, and a family member consistently responded favorably to thyroid therapy. Their depression resolved.

An outstanding case was one of my close friends who came to me for treatment of his pain. A thorough history revealed severe depression with suicidal tendencies. Antidepressants failed to diminish the depression, and he was ready to throw in the towel. He had always been happy and productive in his younger days. Now, his work performance was suffering, and his social life nonexistent. The dry puffy skin, cold hands and feet, chronic pain, low basal temperature, and positive family history for thyroid related illnesses made the diagnosis of hypothyroidism obvious. Proper treatment over a period of two years resolved most of his symptoms including the depression. We enjoyed a tearful embrace when he told me of his marriage plans and great happiness with life.

Seasonal affective disorder (SAD) describes patients who suffer depression only during the winter. Dr. Ord's treatise on myxoedema (the Irish and British spelling) stated, "Sufferers from myxoedema have all their symptoms aggravated and suffer from great weakness and depression when exposed to cold. Experience shows that, even while reaping so great a benefit from the use of thyroid, we are still bound to shield our patients as far as possible from exposure to cold."[7]

Suicide is currently the eighth leading cause of death in America. How many patients suffering from depression (with low basal temperatures and other stigmata of hypothyroidism) would be willing to undergo a trial of thyroid hormones?

Documentation of severe mental problems associated with hypothyroidism began with The Clinical Society of London's Report in 1888. Almost half of the 60 patients from the initial study suffered from delusions and hallucinations, "mainly where the disease was advanced". Insanity was also common in the forms of dementia, melancholia [depression], and acute or chronic mania. Agoraphobia was present in several cases. This neurosis is an intense, irrational fear of open spaces characterized by marked fear of being alone or being in public places.[1] Neuroses of all types, personality disorders, and other severe mental illnesses were well represented in my patients.

One slender 61 year-old female patient of mine had a constellation of Type 2 hypothyroid symptoms including pneumonia as an infant, chronic cold intolerance, iron deficiency anemia following puberty, gray hair in her 20s, severe menstrual bleeding at 40 resulting in a hysterectomy, marked dental problems, and digestive disorders. Following a severe infection at age 33, bouts of depression began. Within several years, episodes of mania developed. She was diagnosed with bipolar disorder and hospitalized several times. Years later, she was diagnosed with Type 1 hypothyroidism and placed on a small dose of Synthroid®, a synthetic thyroid hormone. A history of low blood pressure as well as the severity of her symptoms led to my diagnosis of mild adrenal deficiency in addition to Type 2 hypothyroidism. She had just begun treatment with desiccated thyroid and adrenal hormones, when a manic attack began. An extra dose of adrenal hormones completely reversed the manic attack. She believes, as do I, that her Type 2 hypothyroidism and adrenal deficiency were the underlying cause of her chronic mental illness.

In 1944, Dr. Zondek discussed the coincidence of hypothyroidism and psychotic disorders in the renowned journal *Lancet*. The title of the article was "Myxedema and Psychosis". He said, "Sometimes genuine psychosis of manic or depressive character, with outbreaks of rage or fury, are observed. Other characteristic features are hallucinations of smell, and less often, sight and hearing, delusions of persecution, and clouding of consciousness."[57]

Dr. Zondek also cited the case of a 23 year-old woman who developed hypothyroidism, then schizophrenia after a pregnancy. Initially, she began to gain weight and lose hair. She was admitted to a sanatorium where true schizophrenia was diagnosed by a competent psychiatrist. Fortunately, she was transferred to Dr. Zondek's care at the Bikur Cholim Hospital in Jerusalem. Dr. Zondek stated, "On admission to our department she described her state of mind as follows: I have lost my memory, which used to be excellent. I am tortured by daydreams. Day and night I hear voices talking to me, and I am talking to them. There are machines in my body which compress my throat. I am irritated by an electric current. There is a constant humming in my ears. When people pass me in the street they curse me or make fun of me. I am tormented by bad smells. I always weep, particularly at night, because I am suffering so much. Sometimes I think all these ideas are not real, and sometimes I am convinced they are." She believed that she was under permanent supervision by the government. Her physical exam showed a puffy face with swollen eyelids, rough voice, sluggish movements, dry skin, scanty hair, sluggish reflexes, and her BMR was 28% below normal. She was placed on a relatively large dose of desiccated thyroid hormones. After only two weeks of treatment, all of her psychotic symptoms had disappeared. Her physical symptoms improved as well. Dr.

Zondek stated, "A year after leaving the hospital the patient was still perfectly all right physically and mentally, leading a normal family life and taking full charge of her household affairs."[57]

I attempted to treat one 40 year-old patient with chronic schizophrenia for hypothyroidism. He was completely unable to follow the prescribed thyroid therapy and treatment failed. Many of the more severe, long-standing psychoses and personality disorders are refractory to treatment. However, other physical symptoms associated with thyroid deficiency will improve if the hormones are properly administered.

Paresthesias are abnormal sensations such as tingling, burning, or formication (a tactile sensation similar to small insects crawling on skin). These usually occur in the extremities, particularly upon awakening. Many of my hypothyroid patients suffer paresthesias as did I. A number of patients also complain of numbness and cramping in their hands.

Carpal tunnel syndrome has been closely associated with hypothyroidism. However, the vast majority of these patients are never evaluated by a good medical history and physical exam for hypothyroidism.

The tendency to fall is mentioned repeatedly in the historical literature. Dr. Ord's description from his 1901 publication bears repeating, "Her gait presented a distinct ataxic [lack of coordination] quality. As her bulky body moved across a room there occurred at each step forward a quiver running from the legs upwards, such as may be seen in people under the influence of great emotion, as in a Lady Macbeth. This appeared to be due to a want of complete concert in the action of the flexors and extensors of the body, the flexors acting for the most part in advance." He continued, "The gait already described is typical of myxoedema, and the tendency to fall, as mentioned in the first case, usually exists, to the production of many accidents."[7]

Modern textbooks regarding hypothyroidism continue to mention the neurologic and psychiatric effects of the disease. However, without exception, the patients whom I have seen do not receive adequate evaluation or treatment for hypothyroidism.

In the vast majority, the possible link between their psychiatric or neurological problems with hypothyroidism was completely ignored. In a few, investigation ceased due to normal thyriod blood test results.

A prominent medical textbook listing of neurological and psychiatric manifestations of hypothyroidism follows.

Table 8.3
Neurologic and Psychiatric Manifestations of Hypothyroidism

Neurologic Symptoms or Signs
  Headache
  Paresthesias
  Carpal tunnel syndrome
  Cerebellar ataxia [a type of incoordination]
  Deafness: nerve or conduction type
  Vertigo or tinnitus
  Delayed relaxation of deep tendon reflexes

Cognitive deficits: calculation, memory, reduced attention span
  Low-amplitude theta and delta waves on EEG
  Prolonged evoked potentials
  Sleep apnea
  Myxedema coma
  Elevated CSF [cerebral spinal fluid] protein concentration

Psychiatric Syndromes
  Depression: akinetic or agitated
  Schizoid or affective psychoses
  Bipolar disorders

Source: DeGroot, L. J., Larsen, P. R., and Hennemann, P. R. *The Thyroid and Its Diseases*. 6th Ed. New York: Churchill Livingstone, 1996. Table 9-3 pg. 342. Reprinted with permission.

A recent book entitled *Could It Be B12? An Epidemic of Misdiagnoses* is a must read for patients and doctors alike. The entire spectrum of neurological problems and developmental disabilities, in addition to a host of other problems, may result from this common deficiency. Standard blood tests for B12 often miss this problem that I see very frequently among my patients.[100]

Dizziness and Vertigo

Dizziness and vertigo have been repeatedly associated with hypothyroidism in medical texts since The Clinical Society of London's 1888 report. With few exceptions, patients complaining of dizziness in my practice suffered hypothyroidism. Most of these patients were previously diagnosed with Meniere's disease.

Prosper Meniere was a French doctor who described fluctuating attacks of hearing loss as being associated with tinnitus and attacks of dizziness or vertigo. An abnormal accumulation of fluid in the inner ear was thought to be the culprit. Dr. Meniere died in 1862 (30 years before hypothyroidism was first cured).

Twentieth century muscle pain specialists such as Hans Kraus M.D. and Janet Travell M.D. described dizziness resulting from tender knots, often called trigger points, located in the sternocleido-mastoid muscles. These muscles originate just behind our ears (on the bone of the skull) and attach to the collarbone in the midline (the sternum) as well as slightly lateral to the midline (on the clavicle or collarbone).[58,59]

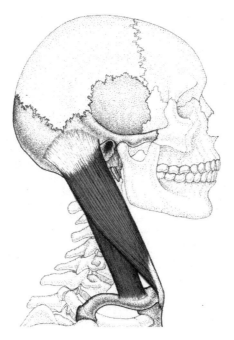

Specialized nerve cells, within the sternocleidomastoid muscles, are named "proprioceptors". These nerve cells send messages to our brains, which allow us to tell what position our head is in when our eyes are closed. This feedback mechanism is dysfunctional in muscles and nerves affected by hypothyroidism. Proper treatment of the hypothyroidism as well as the affected muscles resolves the problem with dizziness in the vast majority of cases.

The Heart

One statement made by Dr. Barnes sticks in my mind, "The first symptom of hypothyroidism a patient may notice could be a heart attack." The illness is insidious. Patients and doctors do not recognize other subtle warning signs such as dry skin or fatigue. Instead, they attribute symptoms to age, or at least they commonly fail to make the connection with hypothyroidism. As previously stated, the rate of heart attacks decreased by 90% in Dr. Barnes' treatment study relative to equivalent patients in the Framingham Study (refer to Chapter 3).

Recall from the section on mitochondria (Chapter 6), "Eventually it became clear that the tissues and organs most readily affected by cellular energy declines [in order of impact] are the central nervous system, followed, in descending order of sensitivity, by the heart and skeletal muscle, the kidneys, and hormone-producing tissues."[34]

The heart muscle is profoundly affected in hypothyroidism. The muscle is infiltrated with mucin, becomes weak, and unable to pump blood efficiently. The medical term for this condition is **congestive heart failure or CHF**. Cardiac output is the amount of blood that is pumped from our hearts. The heart begins to "fail" as the cardiac output drops. Over five million Americans currently suffer from CHF. More than half a million new cases are diagnosed each year. Fifty percent of patients die within five years of their initial diagnosis. Throughout all of my years of formal medical training, not once did I witness the successful treatment of CHF with thyroid hormones. I have since learned to expect resolution of CHF after treatment with desiccated thyroid.

Dr. Zondek was the first to publish a report that linked CHF with hypothyroidism. The following X-rays are from Dr. Zondek's initial report published in a German medical journal from 1918. The enlarged heart is shown to shrink to normal size within weeks of treatment. The patient's symptoms associated with heart failure, as well as hypothyroidism, resolved.[31]

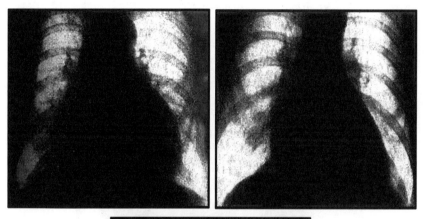

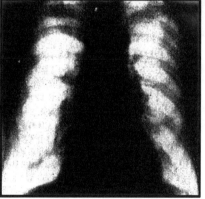

Source: Zondek, H. 1918. The Myxedema Heart. *Munchen Medical WSCHR*. 65:1180.

News of Dr. Zondek's successes spread quickly. By 1925, an article that outlined the diagnosis and treatment of heart failure associated with hypothyroidism was published in *The Journal of the American Medical Association*. George Fahr M.D. stated, "The shape of the heart in severe myxedema is so characteristic that Dr. Rigler, the roentgenologist at the hospital, diagnosed the second and third cases in my series after examination of the roentgenogram [X-ray] alone." He described this characteristic appearance as a heart, "enormously dilated in all chambers." This is the most common form of congestive heart failure (CHF). Normalization of the heart size followed treatment with thyroid hormones. The following X-rays showed the heart's dramatic return to normal size. To demonstrate that the thyroid hormones were responsible for the change, the hormones were stopped for six weeks. The fourth X-ray shows the heart beginning to enlarge. Thyroid hormones were restarted, and the heart size normalized once again.[60]

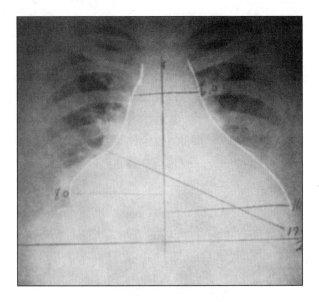

1. Frontal chest X-ray of a 46 year-old woman's heart prior to beginning thyroid. The heart is the large white mass; dark lines are shadows between the ribs. Her BMR (basal metabolic rate) was 25% below normal. Oct. 8, 1923.

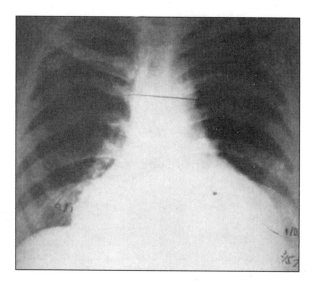

2. Twelve days after beginning thyroid medication, her BMR was 10% below normal. Oct. 24, 1923.

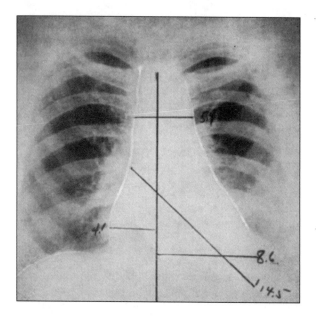

3. Sixty-eight days after beginning thyroid medication, heart returned to normal size. Her BMR was 3% above normal. Dec. 19, 1923.

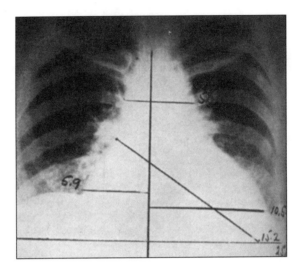

4. Six weeks after thyroid stopped, heart was enlarging again. Her BMR was 10% below normal. Feb. 24, 1924.

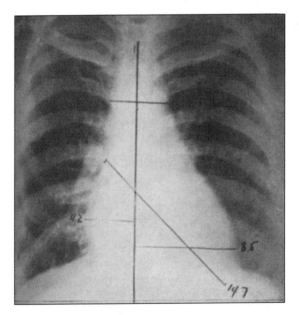

5. Five weeks after restarting thyroid, heart returned to normal size again. Her BMR was 5% above normal. Mar. 12, 1924.

Source: Fahr, G. Myxedema Heart. *JAMA* 1925; 84(5); 345-349. Reprinted with permission.

Renowned modern medical texts on hypothyroidism prominently mention its effect on the heart, "Pulse rate and stroke volume
are diminished in hypothyroidism, and cardiac output is accordingly
decreased, often to one-half the normal value."[54] In other words, the
heart is often markedly impaired. To my amazement, two paragraphs
later, Dr. Zondek's 1918 paper was cited, "The term Myxodemherz
(myxedema heart) was introduced by Zondek in 1918. It embraced
dilatation of the left and right sides of the heart, slow, indolent heart
action with normal blood pressure, and lowering of the P and T waves
of the electrocardiogram. These findings have been confirmed and
extended, and some investigators believe that congestive heart failure
may develop in the absence of other organic cause and may respond
therapeutically to thyroid hormone therapy."[54] This textbook, *The
Thyroid and its Diseases*, was printed in 1996. The successful treatment
of heart failure espoused by Dr. Zondek, Dr. Fahr, and many others
from the first half of the twentieth Century has been neglected for
over 80 years.[54,60]

Dr. Zondek's textbook, *The Diseases of the Endocrine Glands*,
provided the most detailed descriptions regarding the effect
of hypothyroidism on circulation and the heart. Dr. Zondek
addressed the treatment of heart failure due to hypothyroidism in
the following excerpt, "The curative effect of replacement therapy
[thyroid hormones] clearly demonstrates the nature of the cardiac
changes. When thyroid hormone is given, the heart grows smaller
almost week by week. Diminution of the heart's size is seen after 15-
20 mg thyroxine (T4) has been given in the course of three to four
weeks. Ultimately the heart may return to its normal size. This has
been confirmed by Assmann; Curschmann; Meissner; Fahr; Mussio;
Fournier; Means, White and Krantz; Lerman, Clark and Means; H.
Werner; J.M. Lopez Morales; and others. Only the widening of the
aorta [the primary artery from the heart] remains irreparable. It is,
I believe, due to more or less extensive atheroma of the aortic wall;
similar changes have been seen, e.g., in thyroidectomized sheep,
by Von Eiselserg; Pick and Pineles, and others. The characteristic
phenomena are shown in the following case history:"[8]

Dr. Zondek described the case of a 57 year-old laborer. He
had been treated 16 years earlier for rheumatoid pains, attributed

to lead poisoning. The pains frequently recurred during the following years. He developed increased weakness in his legs and had difficulty walking. He had problems speaking, and his voice became slower, deeper, and gruff. He developed problems with tinnitus, and his hearing declined. His arms and legs became increasingly weak and developed clumsiness resulting in falls. He suffered chronic pains in his legs and became breathless climbing stairs. He had not perspired for three to four years and always felt cold, even in the summer. On physical exam, his skin was dry and puffy, especially around the eyes. He had diminished hair on his chest, armpits, and limbs. The pulse was 56 beats per minute and his blood pressure was 180/70. The heart sounds were weak and his reflexes sluggish. Dr. Zondek diagnosed hypothyroidism and myxedema heart (heart failure). Patient was treated with thyroid hormones and gradually recuperated. The following X-rays of the patient's chest illustrate the remarkable effect of thyroid treatment on his enlarged heart.

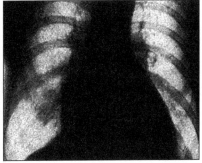

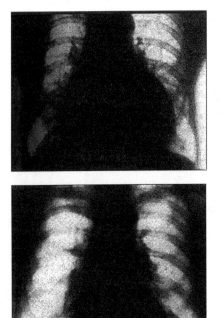

Source: Zondek, H. *Diseases of the Endocrine Glands*, 4th Ed. Baltimore: The Williams and Wilkins Company, 1944. Reprinted with permission.

At age 86, my father chose death instead of undergoing amputation of his right foot and confinement to a wheelchair. He had already lost most of the use of his hands due to rheumatoid arthritis and was dependent on my mother for much of his care. Peripheral vascular disease resulted from decades of untreated hypothyroidism. Dad referred to himself as "The Bionic Man" after a pacemaker placement 10 years earlier. Four years before his death, he suffered congestive heart failure. An X-ray taken during his initial episode of heart failure revealed a heart the size of a volleyball. I will never forget the sinking feeling and churning in my stomach when I saw his X-ray. After four years of proper thyroid therapy, the size of his heart had returned to normal, his coronary arteries were relatively clean, and his heart was pumping blood normally. His doctors could not believe his heart was no longer contributing to his ill health and performed a coronary catheterization and echocardiogram just prior to his death. He died from a hospital-acquired infection (sepsis) following knee replacement surgery.

The heart's electrical system (nerves) also suffers. This weakness is often reflected in the electrocardiogram, also called the ECG or EKG. The EKG is a measure of the electrical voltages of the heart. The resultant low voltage emitted by a weakened heart was almost diagnostic of hypothyroidism according to Dr. Barnes. Dr. Zondek was the first to describe in great detail the effect hypothyroidism had on the electrocardiogram. He outlined treatment and cited numerous cures in his famous textbook.[8]

Conduction difficulties arise from mucin infiltration in the heart muscle and mucin accumulation around its intricate set of nerves. Palpitations, increased or decreased heart rate, preventricular contractions, atrial fibrillation, and other conduction problems are common. Many of my patients suffered frequent preventricular contractions as well as other arrhythmias (irregular heartbeats). Most patients who persevered and finally received adequate dosages of desiccated thyroid saw their heartbeats normalize.

Watery effusions may accumulate around the heart (pericardial effusions). Dr. Zondek stated, "In 7 out of 22 sheep that had been rendered artificially myxedematous, Goldberg found pericardial effusion. In man such extreme cases of vascular permeability for water occurs but rarely."[8] Pericardial effusions have markedly increased during the last 75 years since his text was first published.

Angina, a suffocating type of chest pain, was as rare as pneumonia in Dr. Barnes' treated patients. He discusses this in his book, *Heart Attack Rareness in Thyroid Treated Patients*, which was published in 1972. Yet, Dr. Barnes' studies remain neglected by cardiovascular doctors 30 years later.[22]

The Lungs

Dr. Barnes believed a case of pneumonia was a strong signal to explore the possibility of hypothyroidism. Pneumonia is a red flag for low immune function. The rise in emphysema and lung cancer, which coincided with the drastic reduction of deaths from infection, has already been noted. He believed these problems were in large part due to the chronic respiratory and sinus infections so prevalent among hypothyroid patients.

Older and modern textbooks remark upon the decreased pulmonary (lung) function that often results from hypothyroidism. Difficulty breathing and air hunger may become pronounced as the disease worsens.

Hypothyroidism increases one's susceptibility to developing asthma. Dr. Hertoghe noted the association with asthma in his 1914 lecture. Environmental illnesses and triggers are usually the immediate cause of the attacks. However, asthma patients almost invariably have low basal temperatures, are susceptible to infection, and have family histories consistent with hypothyroidism. Women are twice as likely as men to suffer asthma. Their asthma is often more severe and more likely to result in death. Minorities and women suffer higher rates of asthma and hypothyroidism.

One of my patients exemplified the severe lung problems that may occur. She was a pleasant woman of over six feet in height who suffered from chronic lung and sinus infections most of her life. Her emphysema was first diagnosed at age 26, five years before she came to me. Questioning revealed that both parents suffered chronic pain, and her aunt and sister were on thyroid medication. Her complaints included fatigue, heavy painful periods, weight gain, dry skin, heat intolerance, depression, other psychiatric problems, recurrent infections, as well as chronic pain. The patient spoke in a husky voice. Her physical exam revealed coarse hair, marked myxedema, extremely dry skin, rapid heartbeat, and diffuse tenderness throughout her muscles. She remained relatively free of sinus and respiratory infections for almost one year following treatment of her hypothyroidism and mild adrenal insufficiency.

A point of interest, regarding this patient's case, was her basal temperature. It was above 98.2 °F and remained so during the following year. I relied on the patient's history, physical exam, and thyroid blood tests to rule out <u>hyper</u>thyroidism. Her elevated temperature was probably due to chronic inflammation in her lungs. The basal temperature test for hypothyroidism is not infallible.

High Blood Pressure, Anemia, Circulation, and Kidneys

A diminution of blood flow to one or both kidneys elevates blood pressure. This was initially demonstrated by gradually clamping off blood flow to dogs' kidneys. The lower the blood flow, the higher the elevation in blood pressure.

Dr. Barnes believed decreased blood flow to the kidneys due to hypothyroidism was the underlying cause of most high blood pressure. **Eighty percent of the patients entering his study group with a prior diagnosis of high blood pressure had their pressures normalize with thyroid therapy alone. Only a few of the study group patients required medications other than thyroid hormones to help control their pressure.** Decreased blood flow, due to narrowing of the kidneys' arteries by atherosclerosis (prior to beginning thyroid hormone), was probably the reason why the high blood pressures persisted in the patients who failed to respond. The findings from the Graz autopsy studies compared with the autopsied patients' medical histories supported Dr. Barnes' conclusion. **Dr. Barnes never claimed he was able to reverse established atherosclerosis. A number of previously listed studies have shown its progression can be halted by correcting hypothyroidism.**

My patients' batting average was similar to Dr. Barnes'. Many of the patients required one or two years of treatment with desiccated thyroid before their pressures fell. Some patients normalized within several months. High blood pressure is affecting an increasingly larger segment of our population and is occurring in younger age groups.

Anemia and iron deficiency are common among my population of hypothyroid patients. Bone marrow is where most of the red blood cells are manufactured. When body temperature is low, the marrow becomes too cool. Red blood cell production may drop precipitously in the affected marrow. Dr. Barnes detailed an excellent example of this phenomenon in one of his books. Normally, the tip of a rat's tail does not produce red blood cells, because the temperature is too low. If the tail is sutured inside the rat's belly where the temperature is much warmer, it produces red blood cells.

As previously stated, peripheral circulation to the extremities (especially the skin, hands, and feet) may decline by 40% or more as a result of hypothyroidism. The decline in the body's circulation is one of the most important factors leading to the myriad associated illnesses.[4]

Iron and vitamin B12 deficiencies may also result from hypothyroidism. An article published in *The Journal of the American Medical Association* (March 27, 1997) by The National Center for Health Statistics, Centers for Disease Control and Prevention studied the prevalence of iron deficiency in America. Findings included: A) 9% of toddlers aged one to two years were iron deficient, and 3% had iron deficiency anemia. B) 9% - 11% of adolescent girls and women of childbearing age were iron deficient, 2% - 5% of this group had iron deficiency anemia.

The percentages of iron deficiency would have been markedly higher if the recommended levels of iron put forth by the Barnes Foundation were applied (refer to Chapter 9). There was an absence of chronic anemia among Dr. Barnes' treatment group.

Decreased output of urine from the kidneys is another frequent finding in hypothyroidism. Many full-grown teenagers as well as older patients that I tested often excrete less than one liter of urine in 24 hours. Again, decreased circulation that results from hypothyroidism doesn't allow the kidneys or each and every one of our cells to properly dispose of waste products. The health of the kidneys and patients suffer.

"Contracting granular kidney" was frequently the stated cause of death on numerous historical cases of hypothyroidism, including the first autopsy by Dr. Ord. "Contracting granular kidney" is an outdated medical expression that describes a shrunken, scarred kidney, which reflects the final stage of kidney failure.

Recall from Chapter 6, the kidney is one of the favorite targets of dysfunctional mitochondria. No cases of chronic kidney failure developed in Dr. Barnes' thyroid treated group. None has developed among my patients on adequate thyroid replacement.

The Liver

The liver is responsible for storing glucose (sugar) during digestion and releasing glucose after the cessation of digestion. Blood sugar begins to drop and death will soon follow if an animal's liver is removed. It is imperative for our bodies to maintain constant glucose supplies. It is the primary fuel used by the brain and central nervous system.

The liver frequently functions poorly in hypothyroid patients. Dr. Hertoghe stated, "There is considerable congestion of the liver, the hepatic [liver] cells secrete badly, while the canaliculi [tubular canals running between liver cells] are compressed."[32]

More than occasionally, results of blood tests in hypothyroid patients show mild elevation of the liver's enzymes. This elevation is indicative of compromised function. These enzyme levels return to normal after treatment unless the patient suffers from a separate disease such as hepatitis.

Excess cholesterol is converted into bile salts in the liver. The bile salts are then eliminated. As hypothyroidism progresses and liver function worsens, many but not all patients' cholesterol levels rise. Dr. Barnes included a chapter entitled "The Demise of the Cholesterol Theory" in his book, *Solved: The Riddle of Heart Attacks.*

Everyone in my medical school class had their cholesterol level checked. I was 35 years-old at the time. My cholesterol level was 160. I attributed the low level to daily exercise and a balanced diet. Seven years later, my level was 240. No change in diet or exercise, however, my symptoms of hypothyroidism were much worse. My level was 150 the last time I checked. The drop was due to correction of my hypothyroidism.

"Prediabetic" is now a frequent diagnosis. These patients store glucose more slowly in their livers and may spill glucose into their urine on a glucose tolerance test. Dr. Barnes treated a number of prediabetics. Their glucose metabolism normalized when put on a course of thyroid hormones. None of my patients has developed diabetes after adequate treatment with desiccated thyroid.

It is the liver where carotene is converted into vitamin A. As hypothyroidism and liver function worsen, patients may develop a yellowish tint to their skin due to excessive carotene build up. Their skin color normalizes with thyroid treatment, unless other liver problems are also present.

Hypoglycemia

Hypoglycemia is a frequent problem associated with hypothyroidism. Hypoglycemia means low (hypo) blood sugar (glycemia). Many of the new patients I see carry snacks in order to avoid the unpleasant symptoms that result from going too long without food. The most common symptoms include headaches, shakiness, sweating, anxiety, panic attacks, rapid heartbeat, fatigue, and weakness.

The liver is responsible for maintaining a constant supply of glucose (sugar) in our bloodstream. The overwhelming majority of hypoglycemia is due to hypothyroidism and the resultant sluggish liver function. No new cases of hypoglycemia developed among Dr. Barnes' study group. A number of his patients complained of the problem before treatment. Their symptoms resolved after proper treatment with thyroid hormones.

My experience is similar. However, many of my patients with more severe hypothyroidism and hypoglycemia often require treatment for mild adrenal and iodine deficiencies in addition to hypothyroidism. Chapter 10 is devoted to the diagnosis and treatment of mild adrenal deficiency.

Dr. Barnes' book, *Hope for Hypoglycemia*, delves into detail with regard to the history, diagnosis, and treatment of hypoglycemia. In the book, a simple and accurate diagnostic test for hypoglycemia, introduced in 1954 by Roberto F. Escamilla M.D., is discussed.[55,61] Dr. Escamilla's test, The Insulin Tolerance Test, begins by drawing a fasting blood sugar, then injecting 0.1 units per kilogram of body weight of regular insulin intravenously. Blood sugar (glucose) levels are drawn at 20, 30, 45, 60, 90, and 120-minute intervals. In normal individuals without hypoglycemia, their blood sugar levels drop to around half the initial level within the first 20 to 30 minutes. No physical or mental symptoms occur. Their blood sugar gradually returns to their fasting level within 120 minutes. In patients with hypoglycemia, a more precipitous and prolonged drop in blood sugar occurs. Mild or more serious symptoms such as bizarre or violent behavior and loss of consciousness are possible. Symptoms resolve within seconds after intravenous glucose is administered. Brain damage or even death is possible without proper medical supervision.

Dr. Escamilla recommended half the normal dosage of insulin (0.05 units per kgm) for patients with adrenal deficiency. These patients are much more prone to severe hypoglycemia and more sensitive to insulin. Doctors should heed these precautions if they plan to use this test, as adrenal deficiencies are becoming much more common.

Dr. Barnes believed a good history and physical exam made the diagnosis of hypothyroidism and the hypoglycemia that often resulted obvious. He rarely used the "insulin tolerance test" after his initial research. Teaching doctors to better recognize and treat hypothyroidism would eliminate the need for a tremendous amount of laboratory testing or other expensive procedures and tests.

The Gallbladder

"Fat, female, and 40" (years) is the pneumonic taught to medical students, which represents the typical presentation of gallbladder disease and gallstones. In my experience, this scenario is also a typical presentation of hypothyroidism. Many of my patients' histories included gallbladder disease.

Dr. Hertoghe referred to the generally feeble nature of the linings or endothelial tissues of the gallbladder and urinary bladder associated with hypothyroidism, "They are shed prematurely, and such cavities as the gallbladder and also the urinary bladder are unprotected from the irritating action of their contents." His next reference was to the frequent association of gallstones with hypothyroidism.[32]

A small but significant percentage of hypothyroid patients develop pain that mimics gallbladder disease. The pain occurs around the bottom of the right rib cage in the upper right quadrant of the abdomen. My mother was one such patient. She was diagnosed with classic gallbladder disease on numerous occasions over several decades. She underwent every possible test including repeated ultrasounds and endoscopic exams. No gallstones or abnormalities could be found. At least one surgeon advised removing the gallbladder despite the absence of findings. Her pain finally resolved after treatment for hypothyroidism. After her pain resolved, I learned from the Barnes Foundation that the symptom was associated with hypothyroidism.

The Bladder

From Dr. Hertoghe's lecture, "The bladder being constantly denuded of its epithelial lining is more than usually sensitive to the irritating action of the urine, and this alone is responsible for many cases of nocturnal enuresis (bed-wetting) in children." Dr. Hertoghe also mentioned infections associated with the urinary tract, i.e. bladder and kidneys. Bladder and kidney infections are common in hypothyroidism, especially among women.[32]

Does irritable bladder syndrome and urinary frequency ring a bell? Reason also suggests a significant percentage of bladder cancer may be due to this chronic irritation, coupled with diminished immunity as we age.

The Digestive Tract and Eating Disorders

Starting with the esophagus and ending in the rectum, digestion slows, and its associated secretions are diminished. Problems associated with swallowing, the esophagus, stomach, intestines, and absorption frequently develop. Reflux of stomach acid and ulcers may result. Cancers of the gut are more likely to occur.

Muscle lines the digestive tract including all 28 feet of our intestines. These muscles, their nerves, and blood supply all suffer in hypothyroid patients. Normal digestion requires a huge blood supply. There are as many nerves in the digestive tract as the spinal cord. The gut's nervous system even has its own name, "the enteric nervous system". It is no wonder we feel so badly when our digestive tract is impaired.

Dr. Hertoghe stated, "The scanty intestinal secretion along with the muscular weakness of the visceral walls causes obstinate constipation, which in turn leads to fermentation with the formation of an abnormal quantity of gas, thus producing meteorism [gas in the stomach or intestines] and abdominal distention with noisy eructations from the stomach."[32]

Constipation and excess gas are among the most common illnesses of today. Fecal impaction due to obstinate constipation is not uncommon in the elderly. Constipation usually improves or resolves within several months of proper thyroid therapy.

One-third of my pain patients suffered constipation, often since childhood. The following case study and pictures illustrate the dramatic effect desiccated thyroid hormones can have on the gut.

A 45 year-old woman complained of weakness, sore and stiff joints, slowing of mental and physical activity, impairment of memory, slowing of speech, dryness of skin, lack of perspiration, cold intolerance, some loss of eyebrows and body hair, increasing constipation, and menorrhagia (heavy periods). She also had an accumulation of fluid in her abdominal cavity (ascites), anemia, yellowish skin (carotinemia), an enlarged heart, and a BMR of minus 41%.

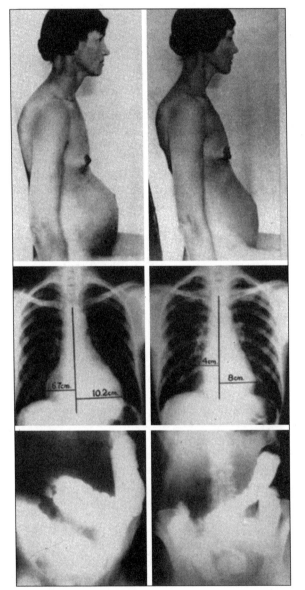

Before treatment   After treatment

Source: Lisser, H., and Escamilla, R. F. *Atlas of Clinical Endocrinology: Including Text of Diagnosis and Treatment*. C.V. Mosby Company, 1957. Reprinted with permission.

The patient's appearance before and after three months of therapy demonstrates resolution of the abdominal fluid (ascites) (figure 5a and b), normalization of heart size (figure 5c and d), and markedly improved colon tone (figure 5e and f). Her periods normalized and her heart rate increased from 51 to 84 beats per minute.[21]

To my knowledge, *The Atlas of Clinical Endocrinology* contains the only description of this variant form of hypothyroidism. The authors named it "internal myxedema" or the Escamilla-Lisser Syndrome after themselves. This case resembles a number of very ill hospitalized patients for whom I once cared. The diagnosis of hypothyroidism was not considered for this constellation of symptoms during my formal training in medical school and residency.

Inflammatory bowel diseases such as colitis were not uncommon in my patients and their families. Diverticulosis may result from hypothyroidism.

Poor appetite and eating disorders such as anorexia may occur. The patients I have seen with histories of eating disorders all suffered from hypothyroidism. I am fond of medical programs on Public Broadcasting Stations. In 2001, a program on eating disorders aired. It showed a significant number of the unfortunate sufferers and their mothers sharing the characteristic appearance of hypothyroidism.

Dr. Eugene Hertoghe stated, "In severe thyroid inadequacy, there is absolute want of appetite, and the aversion for food is unconquerable. Meat is especially distasteful."[2]

Paradoxically, the appetite may be greatly increased. Many hypothyroid patients' hunger is never satisfied. Critical areas and supportive structures in the brain become impaired. Basic bodily functions in addition to mental functions are often affected. The appetite may begin to normalize after lengthy treatment. In his landmark textbook, Dr. Zondek referred to the "obese type" of hypothyroidism as its own entity or subtype of the illness. Refer to the section on obesity for additional information.[8]

Menstrual Disorders, Fertility, and Menopause

The thyroid gland was once nicknamed "the third ovary". Before the twentieth century, women usually began menstruation at the age of 12 or 13. Their cycles would occur every 26 to 30 days and menstrual blood flow would last four or five days. Today, the hypothyroid epidemic has turned the natural cycle into a monthly crisis far too frequently. Profuse bleeding, severe cramps, and other premenstrual problems such as irritability and headache are now commonplace. Endometriosis, fibroid tumors, and ovarian cysts have increased in frequency. All are associated with hypothyroidism. Other hormonal dysfunctions, such as disturbances in estrogen and progesterone, often occur as a result of hypothyroidism and iodine deficiency.

Forty percent of women seen in my pain practice had prior hysterectomies because of the constellation of aforementioned problems. Dilatation and curettage of the uterus was also commonplace. Many of the premenopausal women had severe problems with PMS, profuse bleeding, irregular menses, spontaneous abortions, complicated pregnancies, fibroids, endometriosis, ovarian cysts, and numerous other symptoms.

Dr. Hertoghe stressed the effect of thyroid on menses, "The excessive bleeding is caused by the infiltration of the uterine mucous lining, by the defective contractility of the uterine muscular cells and by the hemophilic condition of the blood." The infiltration to which he referred is the abnormal accumulation of mucin in hypothyroidism. He continued, "The thyroid has a great influence on menstruation, pregnancy, lactation, and even uterine involution after childbirth. We often see women who at ordinary times have a decent supply of thyroid secretion run short during the menses. A large quantity of thyroid stuff is wanted during the menses."[32]

Dr. Barnes published his first paper about the relationship between hypothyroidism and menstrual disorders in 1949. Menstrual cramps of 35 out of 48 women were completely relieved with thyroid hormones. Eight improved and only five failed to get some relief. Of the 45 women who had irregular cycles, 41 normalized, 2 improved, and only 2 were not helped. Of the 50 patients who suffered excessive bleeding, 46 normalized, 2 improved, and only 2 failed to benefit from thyroid treatment. Many of these women stopped their thyroid hormones after their symptoms disappeared. They usually sought Dr. Barnes' help once again after their symptoms recurred. I am happy to report similar results, especially when liberal dosages of iodine are given.[4,62,99]

Historically, perpetuation of the species through reproduction is the most important physiological function imparted to each and every living thing. One in five American couples reportedly now have problems conceiving. Infertility specialists have declared it a disease unto itself. Miscarriages and fertility problems are a red flag for hypothyroidism.

Infertility rates in males are fast approaching those found in females. Sperm banks report a marked drop in the average sperm count of donors during the last 20 years. Impairment of fertility in both men and women because of hypothyroidism is firmly entrenched in medical literature. Whole families disappeared in goiter regions due to impaired fertility. It is also well established that most hypothyroid people are able to reproduce. Widespread pollutants and hormone-mimicking synthetic chemicals also may impair thyroid metabolism and fertility (refer to Chapter 12).

With few exceptions, the patients I have seen with fertility problems, suffered hypothyroidism. Yet, modern texts continue to refute hypothyroidism as a major cause of infertility and miscarriages. Again, the main problem is that affected women and men usually have normal thyroid blood tests.

In 1914, Dr. Hertoghe stated, "We may assert that thyroid extract has proved in scores of cases an excellent remedy for otherwise inexplicable sterility." Dr. Barnes' chapter, "Menstrual Disorders, Fertility Problems, and Avoiding Needless Surgery," provided additional research and medical journal references supporting the efficacy of thyroid hormones in the treatment of infertility. A growing number of my patients have become pregnant after failing expensive and painful fertility treatments.[4,32]

In America, a 27% rise in premature births has occurred during the last 20 years. Twelve percent of all births are now premature. Premature babies have a substantially increased risk of problems related to the central nervous system (the favorite target of hypothyroidism) such as mental retardation, cerebral palsy, and learning disabilities. Current doctrine states the number one risk factor for premature births is already having had one. In my opinion, the leading cause is Type 2 hypothyroidism.

A 2001 PBS television special about infertility featured a plethora of clearly myxedematous mothers. Recently, I also saw a picture of the first test tube baby, now grown. She, too, has the typical appearance of the obese form of hypothyroidism. The offspring resulting from fertility specialists will likely suffer just as many or even more health problems than their mothers, if not given treatment for their hypothyroidism.

During or after a pregnancy, hypothyroidism also causes many problems such as gestational diabetes, high blood pressure, eclampsia (convulsions and coma associated with pregnancy), prolonged labor, inability to dilate, excessive bleeding, poor wound healing, and the inability of the mother to lose weight afterwards.

Dr. Ord described possible effects on pregnancy. Severe post-partum hemorrhages were one sign. He stated, "Pregnancy may occur after the full establishment of the disease, and, as already noted, hemorrhage is to be dreaded. In connection with pregnancy, fluctuations in the swelling of the body may occur. There is sometimes an increase, more commonly a decrease, so that in the early stages the patient may resume almost a natural appearance during pregnancy."[7]

Complications associated with pregnancies were almost nonexistent among Dr. Barnes' patients. He stated on his lecture tapes that only one patient suffered eclampsia. Her first visit to his office was one week before she delivered. She had not been on thyroid therapy long enough for it to help.

I have seen many women who developed pain in and around their C-section or hysterectomy scar. Invariably, these women endured numerous exploratory and imaging procedures such as laparoscopies or MRIs in vain attempts to find the source of their pain. The trouble lies in their muscles and scar tissue, which have not healed properly due in large part to hypothyroidism.

Severe mental and physical problems associated with menopause are becoming commonplace. The onset or worsening of hypothyroid symptoms often coincides with menopause. Dr. Barnes stated that his female patients (taking thyroid hormones) suffered very few symptoms during menopause. Like its effect on puberty, the onset of menopause may be delayed or occur prematurely in hypothyroid patients.[10]

Symptoms also include decreased libido in both men and women. Erectile dysfunction often results. Men's testes may become smaller and softer. One male patient of mine had atrophy of his penis.

Women's genitalia and pelvic organs often suffer severe problems such as atrophy as they age. Pelvic reconstruction surgeries to repair atrophic tissues are common. The women I have seen who have had pelvic reconstructive surgery also suffered hypothyroidism. My mother almost died after suffering a chronic, low-grade, allergic reaction to the plastic mesh that was used for her pelvic reconstruction. Her life was saved by two additional surgeries and treatment for her allergy by environmental medicine specialists. The breasts are usually much less affected than the pelvic organs.[8]

Chronic Fatigue Syndrome

Chronic Fatigue Syndrome (CFS) is another mysterious malady characterized by a constellation of symptoms for which multiple causative factors have received blame. Decreased adrenal function and a weak immune system that allows chronic yeast (Candida Albicans) or viral infections to fester are among commonly accused culprits.

Symptoms of CFS in addition to "unexplained" persistent fatigue may include decreased concentration and short-term memory, headaches, muscle and joint pain without swelling and redness, tender lymph nodes, sore throat, unrefreshing sleep, post-exertional malaise lasting 24 hours or more, along with a host of others.

According to our National Center for Infectious Diseases (part of the CDC), hypothyroidism must be ruled out by a TSH blood test. If the patients are already being treated for hypothyroidism, the adequacy of treatment must be verified by a normal TSH blood test. Type 2 hypothyroidism is a cellular problem that escapes detection by standard thyroid blood tests.

In William G. Crook's popular book, *Chronic Fatigue Syndrome and the Yeast Connection*, he quotes a study done by an internist on 1,100 patients who were afflicted with CFS. Eighty percent of the CFS patients suffered recurrent ear, nose, and throat infections as children, acne as adolescents, recurrent hives, anxiety attacks, headaches, and bowel problems later, as well as being unable to tolerate alcohol. Ninety percent of these patients' cholesterol levels were above 225. Over half of these patients returned to their previous health (I am not sure exactly what that means) after being properly treated for chronic yeast infections. These symptoms closely match those of hypothyroidism. Unfortunately, the author does not state his long-term success. My experience with these patients is that many of their symptoms do not resolve or often relapse due to their undiagnosed and untreated hypothyroidism.

I agree with Dr. Crook's contention that chronic yeast infections cause numerous health problems. Yeast infections usually result from repeated courses of antibiotics. Antibiotics wipe out the normal, friendly bacteria in our digestive tract. Yeast is also normally found in the gut. It is usually a friendly helper along with the normal bacteria, which help digest the food we eat. However, the yeast is a fungus, which is not killed by antibiotics. The yeast multiplies and may become a serious health problem for both men and women. Therefore, treating our children's hypothyroidism would substantially reduce the use of antibiotics by bolstering their immune systems. If a ten-day course of antibiotics must be given, then antifungal medicine such as Nystatin should be given for 14 days. Nystatin helps to keep the yeast in check while on antibiotics.

Many patients with multiple chemical sensitivities meet the CDC guidelines for Chronic Fatigue Syndrome. Chemically sensitive patients' weak immune systems are often overwhelmed by numerous airborne and food allergies in addition to environmental toxins. In my experience, these patients usually have personal and family histories consistent with hypothyroidism.

The National Institutes of Health recently reported low doses of adrenal hormones might help chronic fatigue patients. Their doctors must have missed William Mck. Jefferies M.D. book, *Safe Uses of Cortisol,* first published in 1981. The second edition was released in 1996. Low dose adrenal hormones were recommended for chronic fatigue patients in both editions.[63]

My patients who suffer from CFS all require thyroid hormone replacement and iodine/iodide. Chronic yeast infections, allergies, mercury and other heavy metal toxins, magnesium and nutritional deficiencies, and dental problems are also common and must be addressed.

Bleeding Problems and Bruising

Severe bleeding problems that occur among the hypothyroid have been documented in every text on the subject since the first comprehensive report was published in 1888. At that time, The Clinical Society of London reported severe hemorrhages that occurred during childbirth. Severe bleeding from the nose, gums, teeth, and bowels was also common among those affected. They stated, "Hemorrhages appear to be much more common than it was at first suspected."[1]

Modern textbooks continue to mention the clotting difficulties associated with hypothyroidism. The antihemophilic factor is reduced as well as other factors associated with normal clotting. The majority of my patients bruise easily prior to treatment. Prolonged oozing of blood from scratches or cuts is common, especially in the elderly. My patients often report a history of nosebleeds, bleeding after dental work, surgeries, and childbirth.

Conversely, the tendency to form blood clots is increased. As hypothyroidism worsens, the circulation and the rate of blood flow through our veins slows down. Tiny muscles that line every vein to help pump the blood back to our hearts may also become weak. The nerves supplying each muscle and blood vessel are negatively affected. Hypothyroidism causes damage to the linings of our arteries, the end result being atherosclerosis. This injury causes the arterial linings to have procoagulant properties instead of their natural anticoagulant properties. The injured arteries secrete chemically active compounds that may contribute to blood clots as well as atherosclerosis.[17]

The resultant impedance in blood flow promotes formation of clots in the deep veins. Blood clots are common in large veins following surgeries for arthritis, heart problems, and other illnesses related to hypothyroidism. "Coach Class Syndrome" has recently gained recognition on airplane flights. Increasing numbers of blood clots are occurring in airline passengers after long flights. Passengers are encouraged to stand and walk more frequently.

The hormones in birth control pills interfere with the proteins that transport thyroid hormones through our blood (thyroid binding globulins). As a result, birth control pills may exacerbate hypothyroidism. Birth control pills are associated with an increased incidence of blood clots and stroke. Dr. Barnes treated a number of women who previously suffered blood clots while on the pill. He believed the reason they suffered blood clots was that they had untreated hypothyroidism. Many hypothyroid patients of mine were unable to take birth control pills due to numerous untoward side effects.[4]

Autoimmune Diseases

Autoimmune illnesses such as lupus and rheumatoid arthritis are linked to hypothyroidism. No new cases of lupus developed in any of the thousands of patients Dr. Barnes treated with thyroid hormones.

Dr. Barnes treated a number of patients who had previously contracted lupus. None of these patients developed any new evidence of internal organ involvement while undergoing treatment with thyroid hormones. Lupus patients often suffer kidney and nervous system damage. Lupus is much more common in women, blacks, and American Indians, as is hypothyroidism.

An article was published by German scientists in the journal *Nature Genetics* (June, 2000). The study indicated an intracellular enzyme's failure to mop up dying cells in mice resulted in their developing lupus.

The cleansing of cellular debris and increased activation of enzymes are among the main functions of thyroid hormones. Most of the connective tissue diseases, including rheumatoid arthritis, polymyositis, amyloidosis, and lupus, are associated with the deposition of mucin in the connective tissues. Deposition of mucin in connective tissues is the hallmark of hypothyroidism.

In 1888, the report from The Clinical Society of London described hypothyroid symptoms involving the face. The report stated, "The features are broad, puffy, and coarse. The eyelids are always the seat of transparent swelling, and the eyebrows are generally raised in order to help sustain the upper lid. The nostrils are swollen and broadened; the lower lip thickened, everted and livid; the mouth widened transversely. Over the cheeks and nose there is a well-defined red patch, in strong contrast with the pallid, porcelain-like orbital area."

In that last sentence, the committee described the characteristic "butterfly patch" on the face, which is typically found in many lupus patients. Thus, the association of lupus with hypothyroidism was noted in the 1888 report. However, lupus had yet to be recognized as a disease. The kidneys and nervous systems are favorite targets of Type 2 hypothyroidism and lupus. A number of my patients initially suffered the characteristic butterfly patch. Often, their doctors had put them through every possible test in vain attempts to make the diagnosis of lupus. Just as Dr. Barnes stated about his patients who were put through the ringer, "The diagnosis of hypothyroidism was written all over their faces."[10]

My father had excellent health until the age of 60. He had taken desiccated thyroid hormones for years. The prescribing doctor told him the hormones would be necessary for the remainder of his life. Unfortunately, the thyroid was stopped after a move and change in doctors. The new doctor said a blood test (TSH) showed he no longer required the hormones. Within a year, my father developed crippling rheumatoid arthritis.

William J. Rea M.D. and other environmental medicine pioneers firmly established an environmental link in numerous cases of autoimmunity. Dr. Rea and the staff at his clinic, The Environmental Health Center of Dallas, have repeatedly reversed one particular form of autoimmune illness known as "Idiopathic Thrombocytopenic Purpura" or ITP. The body begins destroying its own platelet blood cells. Platelets are in large part responsible for the clotting of blood. If there are too few, people hemorrhage and often die. Dr. Rea's clinic is environmentally sterile. The patients are sheltered from pollutants and fed food and water free of chemicals while their environmental illnesses are being treated. Dr. Rea writes about their illness, treatment, and outcomes in the four volume texts entitled *Chemical Sensitivities*.[40,41,67,78] A brief overview of Dr. Rea's work and chemical sensitivities is described in Chapter 12.

The mercury and silver used in dental fillings have both been shown to cause autoimmunity in a strain of mice.[64] One of my patients, who was a dental technician, developed multiple sclerosis (MS) shortly after beginning treatment with thyroid hormones. She had not yet reached a therapeutic dosage. I found high levels of heavy metals such as mercury in her system. After reaching a therapeutic dosage of thyroid and beginning a physiological dosage of adrenal steroid and iodine, her MS has not progressed. Adrenal deficiency is discussed in Chapter 10. Heavy metals' deleterious health effects are discussed in Chapter 12.

Headaches and Migraines

Almost 30% of my patients suffered headaches and migraines. Many doctors specialize in the treatment of headaches, and there are numerous clinics specifically for the treatment of headaches. There are scores of different categories and types of migraines. Wide variations of treatment are recommended.

After realizing the pervasiveness of hypothyroidism, every migraine patient seen in my clinic was affected with the illness in my opinion. Many of the patients had additional problems such as estrogen and progesterone deficiencies, adrenal dysfunction, chronic Candida (yeast) infections, heavy metal toxicity, chemical sensitivities, or environmental allergies.

One such patient was a friend of mine and was desperate for help. The unfortunate fellow suffered a particularly nasty form of migraines called cluster headaches. They began suddenly following a car accident 15 years earlier. The cluster headaches recurred every 12 to 18 months without any apparent precipitating cause. Torturous headaches persisted for periods of two to three months and suddenly disappeared.

High dose prednisone often shortened their course. My friend contemplated suicide due to the severity of pain. The MRI of his brain, electroencephalogram, and spine X-rays were all unrevealing. Standard tests such as these are almost always negative when searching for the underlying cause of headaches. My friend had a history of boils, sinus problems, and suffered high blood pressure from an early age. He was overweight and felt hot the majority of the time. His feet were cool and dry, skin and eyes quite puffy, nails ridged and discolored, and his left great toenail was removed "because it curled under." His only sibling was a sister who died of a brain tumor at the age of six. His mother died at 76 from colon cancer, and his father had his first heart attack at age 70. It has been seven years since his last migraine. He takes 4 grains of desiccated thyroid daily.

Several major muscle groups around the head and neck receive their nerve supply from the same nerves that innervate our senses. These nerves are called the cranial (head) nerves and are responsible for smell, vision, hearing, taste, sensation of the face, and other critical functions noted earlier. The cranial nerves have a complicated system of interconnections between themselves. It should not be too surprising that when these muscles and the cranial nerves are infiltrated with mucin, headaches may result. The blood vessels and linings of the nerves that nourish the brain can be infiltrated by mucin, as can the supporting tissues within the brain itself.

Many patients report difficulty taking their rings off, and their shoes may be too tight at the onset of a migraine. Excess fluid retention can often be attributed to the compromised circulation associated with hypothyroidism. Tissues within the skull also swell and migraines result. Bed-rest often allows the excess fluid to be excreted and the migraine to resolve.

The dura mater is the outermost covering of the brain and spinal cord. Interestingly, the ganglion or nerve cell body of the fifth cranial nerve (trigeminal) is located between the two layers of the dura mater below the base of our skull. Among other things, this critical body of nerves transmits data for pain, temperature, and touch from the extensive area of distribution that the nerve supplies. This particular nerve is responsible for the sensation of our skin including the face and forehead, nearly all of the scalp, our oral and nasal cavities, paranasal sinuses, teeth, muscles used in chewing, and contributes sensory fibers to most of the dura mater. Tic douloureux is a pain syndrome involving the trigeminal nerve. It is an extremely painful condition, and its cause is unknown. The few patients I have seen with tic douloureux suffered the typical stigmata of hypothyroidism.

Headaches associated with the menstrual cycle were "classic symptoms" of hypothyroidism according to the senior Dr. Hertoghe. My female patients who suffered migraines often associated them with their menstrual cycles.

Dozens of very sick patients of mine with long horror stories of migraines have histories of sinus infections and other stigmata of hypothyroidism. Many have undergone repeated sinus surgeries in vain attempts to resolve their headaches. Of course, there are many other possible causes for headaches, such as infections, metabolic disturbances, tension, and trigger points in the musculature of the head and neck. However, most of these additional causes also may result from hypothyroidism.

Dr. Barnes devoted a short chapter to headaches and migraines in *Hypothyroidism, the Unsuspected Illness*. He noted that 95 of the first 100 patients he treated for migraine responded well to thyroid therapy alone.[4]

Chronic Pain, Arthritis, and Fibromyalgia

Drs. Kraus and Sonkin attributed chronic, diffuse pain to underlying endocrine problems. They regarded the diagnosis of fibromyalgia with disdain. It is curious to note that the fibromyalgia syndrome began to attract attention in the 1970s. During the 1970s, the vast majority of doctors began treating patients with synthetic thyroid (T4) instead of desiccated thyroid. The latter half of the twentieth century was also when treating thyroid blood tests instead of treating patients' symptoms became the accepted standard. Chapter 9 is devoted to an explanation of the various treatments of hypothyroidism throughout the history of the illness.

Muscle cramps were frequent among my pain patients. Muscle cramps are prominently mentioned in a 1974 book authored by Dr. Ian Ramsay, "Thyroid Disease and Muscle Dysfunction." He estimated that about half of patients with hypothyroidism suffered muscular pain.[36]

Dr. Barnes included a chapter on arthritis in his book about hypothyroidism. He noted the great similarity of symptoms shared by both arthritic and hypothyroid patients. Dr. Barnes also cited research published in 1929 by Dr. Loring Swaim from Harvard. The doctor noted the obvious similarities between patients stricken with arthritis and those suffering hypothyroidism. BMR testing demonstrated lower than normal metabolism in a majority of cases. Dr. Swaim treated all of the affected patients with thyroid hormone with mixed results. Once certain disease states begin, they are often difficult to reverse.[65]

The basal metabolism test results for my pain patients were much lower on average than those performed by Dr. Swaim in 1929. Many of my patients showed no evidence of arthritis. However, abundant evidence of hypothyroidism and other hormone deficiencies were conspicuous, especially among my arthritic patients.

I abandoned the BMR after discovering Dr. Barnes' book. Since that time, the basal temperature test has indicated hypothyroidism in all but a few pain patients. Dr. Barnes stated the effects of pain and inflammation on a small number of arthritic patients may falsely elevate their temperatures and basal metabolism.

Dr. Hertoghe's lecture from 1914 included detailed descriptions regarding the infiltration of muscle cells with mucin and fat. The infiltration was "accompanied by stiffness and dread of movement." He continued, "The connective tissue sheath which supports the contractile elements and connects the muscles with the tendons, and articular ligaments is equally infiltrated, and this adds to the difficulty of movement."[32] He noted the effect applied to both voluntary muscles as well as smooth muscles contained in the blood vessels, bladder, and intestines. The infiltration also affected cartilage.

> "On moving the joints which are stiff and painful, the application of the hand detects a peculiar sensation resembling the crackling of crushed snow which is almost pathognomonic [diagnostic of hypothyroidism]. This is well felt in the knee joint." Dr. Hertoghe had just given a perfect description of one of the first signs doctors are taught to look for when diagnosing arthritis. "These painful affectations of the joints improve very slowly and are the last symptoms to disappear."[32]

Articular rheumatism was the term applied to joint pain in the early twentieth century. At the time, the recommended treatment was thyroid extract. Accelerated arthritis, joint effusions, bone infections, as well as fractures that fail to heal are all signs of hypothyroidism. The most severe osteoporosis I have seen involved elderly chronic pain patients who received prednisone for pain and arthritis either constantly or periodically for years. Osteoporosis is another long-term complication of hypothyroidism. The fact that prednisone inhibits thyroid metabolism and worsens hypothyroidism is discussed in Chapter 11.[66]

Younger and younger patients are undergoing joint replacements due to the increasing severity of osteoarthritis, the most common form of arthritis. Friends and patients who underwent operations in their 40s and early 50s bear family histories and symptoms consistent with Type 2 hypothyroidism.

My personal and professional experience in the treatment of chronic pain leaves no doubt that environmental toxins and illnesses contribute a significant percentage to this growing problem. Environmental toxins are discussed in Chapter 12.

Table 8.4

Manifestations of Hypothyroidism in the Skeletal System

Clinical Symptoms and Signs
    Arthralgias, joint stiffness
    Joint effusions and pseudogout
    Carpal tunnel syndrome
    Polymyalgia
    Delayed linear bone growth in children

Source: DeGroot, L. J., Larsen, P. R., and Hennemann, G. *The Thyroid and Its Diseases*. 6th Ed. New York: Churchill Livingstone, 1996, Table 9-2 pg. 342. Reprinted with permission.

Cholesterol

Historically, high cholesterol was a red flag for hypothyroidism. The increase in cholesterol is a late manifestation of hypothyroidism in most cases. Dr. Barnes provided extensive research and numerous historical references documenting this fact.[4,23]

Cholesterol is essential for life. Humans manufacture this essential building block of every cell with equal ease from carbohydrates, proteins, or fat. Many vegetarians have elevated levels of cholesterol. Animal fats and eggs are not required to elevate cholesterol. The constant turnover of our cells requires a steady supply of cholesterol.

The liver metabolizes and excretes excess cholesterol through bile. Normal metabolism of cholesterol is often impaired by the compromised liver function that may result from hypothyroidism.

High cholesterol has now become closely associated with premature death by pharmaceutical companies and many doctors. "The Demise of the Cholesterol Theory" is a must read chapter from Dr. Barnes' book, *Solved: the Riddle of Heart Attacks*. In this chapter, he warns of the dangers of polyunsaturated fats.

Dangerous free radicals form when polyunsaturated fats are metabolized. These fats increase the risk of developing cancer.[23]

To further emphasize the influence of thyroid hormones on cholesterol, I will once again show Dr. Sonkin's research on the subject. The following graph illustrates how many of Dr. Sonkin's patients with normal thyroid blood tests responded well to thyroid hormones. One hundred consecutive patients with symptoms of hypothyroidism were tested. The change in basal metabolism and cholesterol levels were plotted on the graph. The patients represented by the darkened circles reported improvement of their symptoms. The patients represented by the clear circles reported no improvement in their symptoms (negative clinical response).

Therapeutic Trials (TSH and/or T-4 normal)

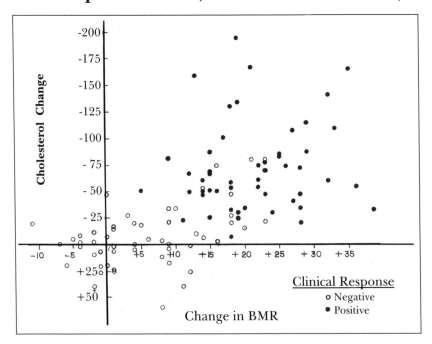

Source: Gelb, H. *Clinical Management of Head, Neck, and TMJ Pain and Dysfunction*. Philadelphia: W. B. Saunders, 1977. p. 162. Reprinted with permission.

The horizontal line represents the change in BMR after a trial of thyroid hormones (a combination of T3 and T4). Two-thirds (66/100) of the patients' BMRs increased from 10% to 35%. The vertical line represents the drop in patients' cholesterol. Following treatment, over half of the patients' cholesterol dropped from 25 points to 200 points. A majority of the patients' hypothyroid symptoms improved.

Pathological studies confirm the sequence of events that occur in atherosclerosis. Tissue damage of the arterial lining occurs first, followed by an accumulation of fat on the lining. The accumulation of cholesterol appears later as the plaque (scar) is formed. The appearance of cholesterol is part of the healing process, not the cause of the damage. Additionally, Dr. Barnes and others have documented autopsy studies from underprivileged countries where heart attacks were scarce. More atherosclerosis was found in the underprivileged children than in Americans. Heart attacks were scarce due to the high rate of deaths from infections. As the incidence of tuberculosis declined in the underprivileged countries as well as in Japan (where heart attacks were more scarce than other Western countries), the incidence of heart attacks rose. Dr. Barnes' autopsy studies from Graz confirmed this finding. The Graz autopsy studies also proved the decline in heart attacks during World War II was due to a rapid rise in deaths from tuberculosis. The population of Graz was deprived of animal fats and cholesterol during the war. Their autopsies showed atherosclerosis accelerated four times as fast than either before the war or years later when plenty of animal fats and dairy were again being consumed.[17,22,23,68]

Not addressing Type 2 hypothyroidism explains why our government and health care providers haven't budged heart disease from its position as the number one killer, despite their massive effort and countless billions of dollars worth of drugs and low fat foods.

Cancer

As previously stated, all of the endocrine glands are negatively affected by hypothyroidism. In addition to thyroid cancer, breast, prostate, and other endocrine cancers were common among my patients' families. Leukemia and brain tumors (benign or cancerous) were not infrequent findings in my patient's family histories. In Graz, where hypothyroidism was endemic, the rate of cancer was the highest in the Western world during the years 1930 through 1972 according to Dr. Barnes' autopsy studies.

The comparison of the changing patterns of death between the years 1930 and 1970 merits reprinting:

Table 8.5 **Disease and Death Rates from the Graz Autopsies**

	Per 1,000 autopsies		
Category	1930	1970	% Change
Heart attacks	6.8	69.0	+915
Emphysema	8.6	40.6	+372
Prostatic cancer	1.8	8.3	+361
Cancer in children	1.2	5.4	+349
Bronchial (lung) cancer	11.0	44.0	+300
Category	1930	1970	% Change
Deaths from infections	426	185	−56
Deaths from malignancies	189	240	+27
Deaths from degenerative diseases	238	343	+44
Deaths from accidents	37	47	+27

Source: Barnes, B. O., Ratzenhofer, M., and Gisi, R. 1974. The Role of Natural Consequences in the Changing Death Patterns. *Journal American of the American Geriatrics Society.* 22:176. Reprinted with permission.

Heart disease and emphysema accounted for 90% of the increase in degenerative diseases. Prostate cancer, juvenile cancer, and lung cancer accounted for 86% of the rise in malignant diseases.

Obesity

Sixty-four percent of U.S. adults are overweight or obese according to the 1999-2000 Centers for Disease Control (CDC) survey. The number of adults who are at least 100 pounds over-weight has quadrupled since 1986. The resultant increase in expected deaths due to the increased incidence of cancer, diabetes, and heart disease associated with obesity will soon overtake those deaths resulting from smoking-related illnesses. Eating habits and lack of exercise continue to shoulder the blame. As noted in Chapter 4, a report from the CDC (March, 2001) found the level of physical activity in America did not change between 1990 and 1998. We have a problem—it's called **Type 2 hypothyroidism**. The "obese form" of the illness has more severe long-term consequences than the form associated with normal weight.

One of the latest syndromes associated with obesity is called "Metabolic Syndrome." According to Dr. Earl Ford from the CDC, "This is just another manifestation of the obesity epidemic that we are seeing in the U.S. along with the sedentary nature of our society." According to the National Institutes of Health's definition, you must have at least three of the following five problems in order to qualify for having Metabolic Syndrome. The syndrome consists of increased abdominal obesity (40 inches in men, 35 inches for women), increased fasting triglycerides (above 150), decreased HDL (good) cholesterol (less than 40), elevated blood pressure (above 130 systolic or above 85 diastolic), and glucose intolerance (elevated fasting blood sugar above 110).[69]

Having three of the five risk factors associated with Metabolic Syndrome increased the risk of developing heart disease by 1.7 times and diabetes by 3.5 times, compared to adults with no risk factors within a period of five years. Having more than three risk factors increased the risk of heart disease by 3.7 times, and the risk for diabetes skyrocketed to 24.5 times the normal risk.

Based on data from 8,800 men and women, Dr. Ford's team estimated 47 million Americans (over 20% of adults) have Metabolic Syndrome. Blacks and Hispanics are at higher risk. Improper nutrition, obesity, inadequate physical activity, and genetic factors are the alleged culprits. The aforementioned CDC report on exercise habits stated that racial differences were minimal.

A 2001 book by Sanford Siegal D.O., M.D., entitled *Is Your Thyroid Making You Fat* lends additional credence to the thyroid epidemic. Dr. Siegal specialized in weight loss. He wrote and asked if I would be willing to be on his referral list after having checked with the makers of Armour® (desiccated) thyroid, because I was one of only several hundred doctors in the country who prescribed the medication. In over 40 years of practice, Dr. Siegal found in treating many thousands of patients that desiccated thyroid was much more effective than synthetic thyroid hormones. Dr. Zondek also reported the superior efficacy of desiccated thyroid over synthetic thyroid hormones in the treatment of the "obese form" of hypothyroidism in his 1926 textbook, *Diseases of the Endocrine Glands*. He had not changed his opinion by the time the fourth edition was published in 1944.

The following pictures from Dr. Eugene Hertoghe's paper are illustrative of the dramatic affect desiccated thyroid can have upon the obese form of hypothyroidism.[2]

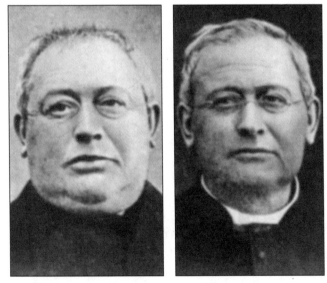

Before treatment   After treatment

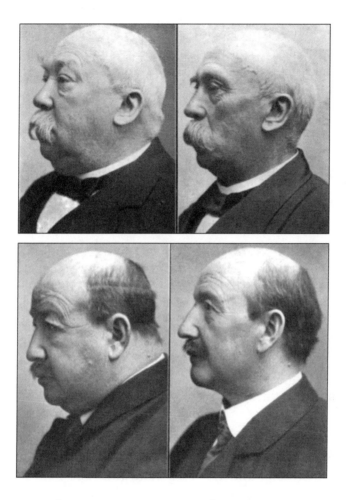

Before treatment   After treatment

Source: Hertoghe, E. *The Practitioner*, Jan 1915, Vol XCIV, No 1, 26-93.

Dr. Barnes' successfully treated himself for hypothyroidism with desiccated thyroid. One of the most intriguing points he emphasized in his lecture tapes and book, *Hypothyroidism, the Unsuspected Illness*, was that a high-protein diet significantly slows down our metabolism. His mentor at the University of Chicago, Anton J. Carlson Ph.D., performed the initial research, which identified that hypothyroid patients' metabolism is already low and that diets high in protein and low in fat compound the problem.

Dr. Barnes illustrated this point by eating a high-protein diet versus a diet high in fat with moderate protein. In order to maintain a constant weight, he consumed three thousand calories per day on the high-fat diet. On the high-protein diet, he was only able to consume two thousand calories. In addition, due to the slower rate of his metabolism, he had to double his dosage of desiccated thyroid hormones to maintain his health. He had developed symptoms of hypothyroidism on the high protein diet. As soon as he switched back to his normal diet, high in fat, he exhibited all of the symptoms of excess thyroid hormone. Within two weeks, he returned to his normal dosage.

> Interestingly, during and after World War II, the vast majority of people in Europe were deprived of eggs and animal fats. Yet, thousands of autopsy results from this period reveal that the rate of atherosclerosis was accelerated to four times the rate before or after this period. Today, the French diet is rich in fat, including lots of saturated fats such as eggs and butter. However, they suffer a lower percentage of heart attacks and this confounds the "experts".

A study from Duke University made headlines in November, 2002. Sixty obese patients were placed on a diet containing 60% fat, high protein, and low carbohydrates (less than 20 grams a day). Another 60 obese patients began the American Heart Association Step One diet: lower in fat (30%) and higher in protein and carbohydrates. The patients lost an average of 30 pounds on the high fat diet compared to 20 pounds on the low fat diet. The high fat diet resulted in an increase of 11% in good cholesterol (HDL) versus no change as a result of the Step One diet. The high fat diet resulted in a 49% drop in triglycerides versus 22% from the Step One diet. Also, patients were better able to follow the high fat diet. Cries of blasphemy and disbelief rang from the mainstream. However, they had no scientific studies to contradict the findings and demonstrate the efficacy of the low fat diet that they had promoted for decades.

Dr. Barnes included a chapter about obesity in his book, Hypothyroidism, the Unsuspected Illness. For decades, he successfully treated hundreds of obese patients with a diet high in saturated fat. Fat allows our blood sugar to remain stable, because it is metabolized slowly and produces a steady stream of calories. This combination helps suppress one's appetite. Patients are not as hungry and lose weight gradually. Carbohydrates are rapidly metabolized, and this results in rapid fluctuations of blood sugar that can stimulate hunger. Dr. Barnes noted numerous other studies that showed high fat diets resulted in more rapid weight loss and more satisfied participants than did high protein diets. On his lecture tapes from the 1970s, he mentioned the superior cholesterol and triglyceride levels associated with the high saturated fat diet versus the high protein diet.

Summary of Symptoms

From Dr. Hertoghe's 1914 lecture, "I need not further multiply examples, but may sum up by saying: When you encounter the association of one or more of the following symptoms: Trophic [degenerative] changes in hair, eyebrows, eyelashes, teeth, or gums; an habitual chilliness, biliary [gallbladder] disturbances with lithiasis [gallstones], dyspnea [labored breathing] with asthmatic attacks; menorrhagia [excessive menstrual bleeding], recurring abortion, hemophilia [prolonged bleeding]; melancholia, depression, weariness of life, migraine, vertigo, sudden loss of consciousness, noises in the ears; somnolence [sleepiness], rheumatoid changes in the muscles, ligaments, or aponeuroses [muscle attachment to tendon]; nocturnal incontinence of urine, pollakiuria [unduly frequent passage of urine], loss of appetite and obstinate constipation-think of a possible deficiency of thyroid secretion."[32]

The effect of declines in cellular energy that results from inheritance of defective mitochondria bears repeating, "Eventually it became clear that the tissues and organs most readily affected by cellular energy declines are the central nervous system, followed, in descending order of sensitivity, by heart and skeletal muscle, the kidneys, and the hormone-producing tissues."[32] Refer to Chapter 6 for details.

Table 8.6

Laboratory Testing for Patients Taking Desiccated Thyroid

1. Instruct patients not to take their desiccated thyroid the morning the test is administered (they may take it afterwards).

2. Free T3 and free T4 usually are within the upper limits of normal if the patients are on the correct dosage of thyroid.

3. The TSH will almost always be suppressed (low) in patients taking two or more grains (> 120 mg) of thyroid. A TSH level of less than 0.01 mIU/L is common.

4. If patients take desiccated thyroid the morning of the test, the free T3 is usually elevated.

Several American labs offer 24-hour urine testing for T3 levels. In America, the current "normal values" or ranges for T3 differ from those utilized by Hertoghe's lab in Belgium (see page 177). Therefore, the American urine tests for T3 remain unproven and inaccurate in my opinion.

Chapter 9
Treatment Guidelines

One of my patients asked why I prescribed hormones since my specialty was pain. I answered, "Because they work!" Prior to training with Drs. Kraus and Sonkin, prescribing hormones for patients never entered my mind. This was the domain of internists, ob-gyn doctors, and endocrinologists. The research and teachings of Drs. Kraus, Sonkin, and Cohen coupled with my own personal experience of being denied treatment due to "normal thyroid tests," opened my eyes. Large numbers of patients were not receiving much needed treatment.

The first successful treatment of hypothyroidism was in 1891. A British doctor, G.R. Murray, cured a case of severe hypothyroidism by injections of animal thyroid gland extract. Later, it was found that beef, sheep, and pig glandular extracts could ameliorate the illness. However, the porcine (pig) thyroid proved to have the most universal efficacy. Desiccated porcine thyroid was mass-produced and remained the predominant form of treatment until the 1960s. Desiccated (dried) thyroid derived from beef and sheep is no longer available. However, they will have to be reintroduced to meet the tremendous need for desiccated thyroid if our population is to receive the best treatment. Also, pharmaceutical companies could manufacture a synthetic duplicate of desiccated thyroid.

In the 1960s, treatment for hypothyroidism took a turn for the worse. Desiccated thyroid lost favor after pharmaceutical companies began to inexpensively mass-produce T4, which is the predominant form of thyroid hormone excreted by our thyroid gland. Nicknamed, "T4," because of the four iodine molecules that are part of its chemical makeup, it was first isolated in 1917 and utilized by university doctors who could obtain limited supplies. The generic or chemical name for T4 is levothyroxine. Pharmaceutical companies patented brand names like Synthroid®, Levoxyl®, and Unithroid™ to market their T4. T4 thyroid hormone is now the only form of thyroid hormone recommended by mainstream medicine and, as a result, is among the most frequently prescribed medicines in the world. However, T4 has relatively little physiological activity and must be converted into T3 in order to be utilized by our cells. Most of the conversion takes place in the liver and kidneys.

T3 contains three iodine molecules and was first produced by pharmaceutical companies in 1949. Since it is thought to have up to ten times more physiological activity than T4, T3 is the principle source of energy for our cells. Sold under the brand name Cytomel®, the manufacturer initially touted T3 as the definitive treatment for hypothyroidism. Its use continues to be promoted by a small minority of doctors.

A research paper entitled, "Why Does Anyone Still Use Desiccated Thyroid USP?" was published in 1978. The pharmaceutical producer of Synthroid® hailed the paper as an endorsement of their patented product. Pharmaceutical representatives encouraged doctors to switch patients from desiccated thyroid to T4, the synthetic thyroid.[71]

The study involved only 40 patients. They were switched from desiccated thyroid to T4 and followed for only six weeks. Six of the 40 patients purportedly showed signs of hyperthyroidism on the initial exam. Five of the six suffered palpitations that may have indicated they were taking too much thyroid. Their palpitations improved or resolved after switching to T4. Aside from these six patients, there was no mention of hypothyroid symptoms either before or after the switching of thyroid hormone. Most of the authors' conclusions were based on thyroid function laboratory tests. In addition, other tests revealed the stated dosages of thyroid hormones were less accurate in the generic desiccated thyroid compared with the synthetic hormone, T4.

The manufacturer of Synthroid® (the brand name for T4) settled a class action lawsuit in the 1990s. There were over 20 recalls due to improper drug dosages. For years, the pharmaceutical company failed to report doctors' complaints of the drug's side effects as required by law. Problems involving the suppression of research on thyroid hormones by a large pharmaceutical company made headlines in *The Wall Street Journal* (04/16/97). Most importantly, **T4 has never been proven to be effective for treating the symptoms of hypothyroidism in any long-term study**. T4 was introduced in 1917, 20 years before the FDA required testing to prove the efficacy of a new drug. T4 is a "grand-fathered" drug, meaning it has earned FDA approval in spite of the fact that its effectiveness was never tested in animal or human studies.

Drs. Cohen and Sonkin frequently used a combination of the synthetic hormones, T4 and T3, in the treatment of their patients. They were not immune to the trend toward synthetic thyroid hormones sweeping over the universities during the twentieth century. As brilliant and ahead of their time as Drs. Sonkin and Cohen were, they did not realize how much more efficacious the desiccated thyroid preparation was than the synthetic hormones.

Dr. Sonkin told me something I would not be able to find anywhere in textbooks, "Patients may display a few symptoms of hypothyroidism as well as a few symptoms of <u>hyper</u>thyroidism simultaneously after the proper dosage of thyroid hormones has been administered." I believe this was due to his use of the synthetic hormones. Desiccated thyroid resolves patients' symptoms much more uniformly.

In Dr. Sonkin's 1997 journal article, one of the families he treated for many decades was mentioned in regard to the high dosages of Synthroid® (T4) they required to overcome their hypothyroidism. The grandfather was taking 0.6 mg, while his daughter was taking 3.0 mg, and her son was on a dosage of 2.7 mg per day. The dosage of 3 mg is about 30 times today's average daily dosage.[56] I asked Dr. Sonkin how he could possibly prescribe so much thyroid medication. His response was, "Because it took that much to wake them up." The patients demonstrated no side effects, and their symptoms markedly improved. In the same article, Dr. Sonkin mentions the fact that the son showed evidence of thyrotoxicosis (an overdose) at 2.9 mg, which necessitated the slight decrease to 2.7 mg in his dosage.

This should serve as a warning not to increase your medication without consulting a physician. These patients received a gradual increased dose over a lengthy period of time and were monitored by a highly skilled endocrinologist.

For the majority of his patients, Dr. Sonkin first administered T4. He would begin with 0.05 mg and increase the dosage to 0.15 mg over several weeks. Next, T3 would be added in 5 mcg increments up to 25 mcg as tolerated. Recall that T3 is the more physiologically active form of the thyroid hormone. After adding T3, Dr. Sonkin stated he would "watch the patients bloom!" Further adjustments in dosages would depend upon the patient's response. Dr. Sonkin treated patients, not lab tests.

After returning from New York to begin a private practice in Missouri in 1996, I began treatment on my hypothyroid patients with Synthroid®. My family and I were also taking the medication. Patients' symptoms improved initially. However, a number of symptoms began to reappear with the passage of time despite increasing dosages well above what most physicians considered "standard". I began adding Cytomel® (T3) to my patients' thyroid medication, as well as to my own. Just as predicted, many patients improved significantly. Again, after the passage of many months, a number of my patients' symptoms of hypothyroidism began to recur.

Dr. Sonkin was consulted once again. He stated that everyone was unique and may require a different combination of the three commercially available hormones (T4, T3, and desiccated). I also asked about my growing population of patients who would not tolerate the smallest available dosage of any thyroid hormones. Many of these patients had low basal metabolic rates in addition to a plethora of the other symptoms and physical findings listed in my chart reviews. There was no doubt in my mind that they were hypothyroid. Other patients only tolerated a small amount before the onset of side effects such as increased heart rate, increased tremor, dizziness, shortness of breath, or chest discomfort.

Drs. Sonkin and Cohen used a thyroid preparation, which was no longer commercially available, in patients who were unable to tolerate the standard thyroid hormones. A derivative of T3 (T3 propionate) that was slowly released into the bloodstream was tolerated relatively well by this patient group. Drs. Sonkin and

Cohen both successfully used the drug, as did Dr. Rawson, Chief of Endocrinology at Memorial-Sloan Kettering Hospital in the 1950s and 1960s.[56]

I contacted a biochemist at the University of Missouri Medical Center, as well as a patent attorney, in the hope of obtaining the drug for my patients. Unfortunately, pharmaceutical companies would be unable to patent the drug because the drug had previously been published in the literature. Pharmaceutical companies do not make as much profit without a patent. There would be no chance of procuring the drug.

Recent publications on the treatment of fibromyalgia advocate the use of a slow-release T3, which is now available through compounding pharmacies formulating bio-identical hormones. Slow-release T3 is apt to cause more side effects than desiccated thyroid. I only use the combination of T4 and T3 in strict vegetarians, patients allergic to pork (porcine thyroid), and for religious preferences. The few patients whom I have seen that were taking T3 for years suffered a number of hypothyroid symptoms as well as having myxedema, the telltale sign of hypothyroidism.

In Dr. Zondek's early text, *Diseases of the Endocrine Glands*, he recognized the superior efficacy of desiccated thyroid, "Thyroiedin [desiccated thyroid] is more efficacious than thyroxine [T4] in the treatment of the obese type of myxedema."[8]

The Barnes Foundation promotes two tenets regarding hypothyroidism. First, the thyroid blood tests fail to diagnose a large percentage of patients. Second, desiccated thyroid is more efficacious than synthetic thyroid hormones.

Dr. Barnes' research on animals and his treatment of thousands of patients over decades proved the superior efficacy of desiccated thyroid. He switched some of his patients to the synthetic hormones as part of his research. Almost all requested to be put back on desiccated thyroid, because they felt better prior to the switch. Dr. Barnes' long-term studies leave no doubt about the efficacy of desiccated thyroid.[4,10,22,23,46,55]

Dr. Barnes performed extensive studies on both animals and humans and determined that desiccated thyroid hormones were far more efficacious than the synthetic hormones, irrespective of the combinations used. During the 1950s, a pharmaceutical company asked Dr. Barnes to test their new product named Thyrolar®. Thyrolar contained a combination of T4 and T3. Twenty percent of his patients who had done well on desiccated thyroid were unable to tolerate the "equivalent" dosage of Thyrolar due to the rapid heart rates or palpitations they developed. Dr. Barnes promptly placed the patients on desiccated thyroid. He suspected that there was something in desiccated thyroid that helped us metabolize the hormones more easily and efficiently.

It appears the old master was right once again. Recent literature supports the existence of other active hormones, such as T2, in desiccated thyroid: "Further transformations to T2 and T1 isomers also occur almost exclusively in peripheral tissue. These transformations are all catalyzed by deiodination (the removal of iodine molecules) enzymes, which remove iodine atoms from the inner tyrosyl or outer phenolic benzene rings. This stepwise deionization is the major route of thyroid hormone metabolism and results in both active and inactive metabolites." **Translation: If a person is unable to convert T4 into T3; T3 into T2; and T2 into T1 (i.e. metabolize thyroid properly), the person's health will suffer.**[79] A recent animal study showed T1 slowed heart rate and induced hypothermia.[101]

In his book, *Solved: The Riddle of Heart Attacks*, Dr. Barnes stated, "I am amazed to see the number of patients who recently have been placed on thyroxine (T4) when the physicians realized that thyroid therapy was needed. Obviously, the patient was not being relieved of the symptoms, or another doctor would not have been sought [Dr. Barnes saw a myriad such patients]. The failure was due to the fact that thyroxine is only a part of thyroid hormone." I concur completely and am happy to report great strides in my patients' health, as well as my family's, after switching to the desiccated thyroid preparation.

Dr. Jacques Hertoghe, the third generation Belgian endocrinologist, worked though the Barnes Foundation to teach American doctors his family's life work. He was one of the principal authors in a long-term medical study concerning the treatment of hypothyroidism that was eventually published in 2001. He and two of his colleagues, Drs. Baiser and Eeckhaut, compared the symptoms of patients already receiving treatment with T4 with a large group of untreated patients who suffered hypothyroidism. Eighty-nine patients with previously diagnosed hypothyroidism had been treated elsewhere with T4 prior to seeking help from these doctors. These patients' symptoms were compared with those of 832 untreated hypothyroid patients who came to their clinic over the same period of time (1984 to 1997). **Symptoms of the patients already taking T4 did not differ from those of the group of untreated patients.**[46]

The 89 patients taking T4 were switched to desiccated thyroid. Symptoms from 40 of the 89 patients were followed for two years. The patients symptoms markedly improved after treatment with natural desiccated thyroid (NDT). The following table illustrates the improvement in eight classical symptoms of hypothyroidism. For example, the prevalence of muscle cramps dropped from 56.2% to 8.7%.

Table 9.1   **Score of Symptoms under T4 and under NDT**

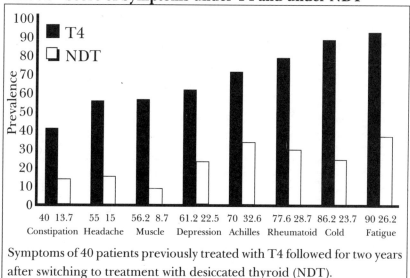

Symptoms of 40 patients previously treated with T4 followed for two years after switching to treatment with desiccated thyroid (NDT).

Source: Hertoghe, J., Baiser W.V., and Eeckhaut, W. Thyroid Insufficiency. Is Thyroxine the Only Valuable Drug? *Journal of Nutritional & Environmental Medicine,* 2001, 11, 159-166. Reprinted with permission.

In addition to those 40 patients, 278 of the 832 previously untreated patients were also monitored for two years. Both groups of patients responded equally well. Prominent hypothyroid symptoms of constipation, headache, muscle cramps, depression, "rheumatoid" (pain and stiffness in joints or muscles), feeling cold, and fatigue were assessed. "Achilles" refers to a delayed reflex involving the "Achilles" tendon at the ankle, another classical finding of hypothyroidism. Following treatment, improvement of patients' symptoms averaged 69% as reflected in the decrease from 10 to 3.6 on symptom scores. The following chart compares the symptoms and laboratory findings between treated and untreated patients.

The 24-hour urine T3 test, introduced by Dr. Jacques Hertoghe in 1984, revealed very little difference between the urine test results from the 89 patients already taking T4 and the 832 untreated patients. Also, there was no difference in the urine tests between the subgroups of 40 and 278 patients who were treated with desiccated thyroid and followed for about two years.

Table 9.2 **Symptoms score and 24 hour urine free T3 in 89 T4 treated patients, of which 40 were subsequently treated with NDT, compared with 832 untreated hypothyroid patients of which 278 were subsequently treated with NDT.**

| | Untreated | | T4 Treated | |
	832	278	89	40
Symptoms score	10.0	10.1	10.4	10.7
Urine T3 pmol	756.0	752.0	767.0	797.5
Months of treatment			38.6	33.2
Thyroxine ug			97.6	99.7
	NDT treated 278		NDT treated 40	
Symptoms score		3.6		3.6
Urine T3 pmol		1900.0		1900.0
Months of ug treatment		23.0		26.9
NDT mg		200.0		233.0

The maximum possible score for symptoms was 16. Pmol (picomol) and ug (microgram) are units of measure. NDT is natural desiccated thyroid.

Source: Hertoghe, J., Baiser, W. V., and Eeckhaut, W. Thyroid Insufficiency. Is Thyroxine the Only Valuable Drug? *Journal of Nutritional & Environmental Medicine* 2001, 11: 159-166. Reprinted with permission.

The approximate "equivalent" dosage of 0.1 mg T4 is one grain (64.8 mg) of desiccated thyroid. The study patients eventually required a dosage from two to five grains of desiccated thyroid. The average dosage was over 200 mg per day (over three grains). These dosages are unheard of in today's medicine. Why? **Because the TSH blood test indicates these patients are all taking too much thyroid. This is just not true. Patients' thyroid glands remain robust (not suppressed) and patients do not suffer ill effects unless they have symptoms of <u>hyper</u>thyroidism or their axillary basal temperature rises above 98.2 °F (normal is 97.8 °F to 98.2 °F).[10] The fact that doctors have been treating misleading blood tests with relatively ineffectual dosages of T4 for over 40 years has resulted in a plethora of erroneous conclusions** (see Chapter 7).

Dr. Hertoghe and his colleagues stated, "It is necessary to stress that the clinical evaluation of a patient's condition must precede interpretation of laboratory tests and not follow it."[46] This concept has historically been paramount in the practice of medicine. The current practice of treating misleading TSH tests and disregarding patients' symptoms and findings on physical exam must stop.

Dr. Barnes' Recommendations

Thyroid must be taken on an empty stomach, at least 20 to 30 minutes before a meal. Dr. Barnes advocated starting with one grain of desiccated thyroid in a relatively healthy adult. He would then add one-half grain one month later and continue to increase the medication every month as needed. Our bodies usually require at least one month to respond to the increased dosage. Dr. Barnes would stop when the patients felt well, experienced any side effects, or reached the dosage of four grains. He occasionally would use five grains, which is the largest size available commercially.

Dr. Barnes recommended one-quarter grain for children under three years. He felt one-half grain was often necessary for children over the age of six. If necessary, one-quarter grain was added every two months in children.

Dr. Barnes advocated a very slow increase of thyroid hormones for patients who had heart disease and a maximum dosage of two grains for anyone with a history of a heart attack. In his studies, heart attack patients were found to be more sensitive to thyroid hormones. He believed heart attack patients should not begin thyroid until two months after their attack. A much smaller starting dose and slower increases proved effective in the victims of prior heart attacks.

One of the lecture tapes available through the Broda Barnes Foundation features Robban Sica M.D. Dr. Sica studied with Dr. Barnes and has specialized in the treatment of hypothyroidism for many years. She stated that patients who had undergone chemical, surgical, or radiation treatments to destroy their thyroid glands (often due to cancer or excess activity) required a minimum of three grains of desiccated thyroid in order to function normally. I agree.

My Recommendations

Adult patients often no longer tolerate the one-grain starting dose of desiccated thyroid that Dr. Barnes recommended. A growing percentage of patients may require therapy for the environmental toxins they harbor prior to beginning thyroid. Toxic chemicals or heavy metals like mercury may block the entire cascade of chemical reactions involved in thyroid metabolism as well as other hormones. The resultant compromised endocrine, nervous, and immune systems contribute to and exacerbate Type 2 hypothyroidism.

Most adult patients tolerate one-quarter to one-half of a grain. For safety's sake, I recommend beginning with one-quarter grain. It is often difficult to ascertain who will be intolerant of the medication. In general, the healthier the patient is, the more likely they will tolerate thyroid. Patients with severe allergies, chemical sensitivities, and chronic pain tend to be less tolerant of desiccated thyroid. These guidelines also apply to Type 1 hypothyroid patients already taking T4 (Levoxyl®, Synthroid®). I treat Type 1 patients on T4 by slowly adding desiccated thyroid, and do not stop the T4 until they are tolerating desiccated thyroid and improving. The stopping of T4 is also gradual. The patients who are intolerant of desiccated thyroid may tolerate T4. Their symptoms often improve by slowly increasing the dosage to tolerance.

For the majority who do tolerate one-quarter grain, I increase the dosage one-quarter grain every 7 to 14 days up to one grain, depending upon the constellation of symptoms, age, and condition of the patient's heart. Gradual increases continue at about one-half grain per month depending on the patient's response. When patients remain symptomatic and show no evidence of side effects, their dosage is increased to four grains before waiting several months in advance of further increases. My patients require an average dosage of three to three and one-half grains, the same dosage the patients in the recent Belgian study required. Some adult patients may only need two grains while others need five. Dr. Sonkin stated in his literature that patients might require as much as 6 to 12 months before responding to thyroid replacement. There is no substitute for clinical experience combined with common sense. Increases or decreases in dosage depend upon patients' responses, blood pressure, heart rates, basal temperatures, Achilles reflex, and a host of other factors. The number one sign of intolerance is an increased heart rate more than 10 or 15 beats per minute above the baseline. Occasionally, patients require larger dosages in spite of an increased heart rate.

A red flag for mild adrenal deficiency, iodine deficiency, or environmental toxicity is a worsening of hypothyroid symptoms as the thyroid dosage is gradually increased. Less fatigue and symptomatic relief is the expected response. Stop or decrease the dosage of thyroid and address these problems should they occur. Chapter 10 covers adrenal deficiency in detail.[63]

At the 2002 Barnes Foundation meeting, Therese Hertoghe M.D., the fourth generation Belgian endocrinologist, expressed her belief that the potency of desiccated thyroid hormones had declined about 50% during the last few decades. Her patients now require larger dosages than her grandfather and great grandfather prescribed. I believe the increased hormone requirement is a reflection of the increased severity of hypothyroidism with each successive generation. The cumulative burden of defective mitochondrial DNA must be a contributing factor. Dr. Barnes predicted the severity of the illness would worsen with each untreated generation. Other doctors associated with the Barnes Foundation agree. Environmental medicine doctors believe the increased burden of environmental toxins is the underlying cause for the precipitous decline in our population's health (refer to Chapter 12). Environment toxins interfere with thyroid and other hormone functions. Our increased burden of genetic defects and environmental toxins must share the blame.

In heart attack patients, a slower increase in dosage is necessary due to the increased work load placed upon the injured heart. Blockages in the arteries feeding the heart can result in chest pain or even a heart attack if the dosage is increased too rapidly. Therefore, two months after a heart attack, I recommend starting patients on one-quarter grain and gradually increasing the dosage, every four to six weeks, until the symptoms improve or upon reaching two grains. A number of doctors associated with the Barnes Foundation believe that it is safe to very cautiously raise the dosage above two grains (2.25 to 2.5) in some heart attack patients. I agree as long as caution and patience are the rule. In addition, frequent monitoring by the patients of their blood pressure and heart rate is necessary.

Patients suffering high blood pressure occasionally need a slower than normal increase of their dosage, similar to the regimen recommended for heart attack patients. High blood pressure may elevate even further if too much thyroid is given too soon. There is no limit on the final dosage unless they have had a heart attack.

It is much easier and more prudent to treat the younger, healthier hypothyroid population. The fact that children respond to treatment for hypothyroidism more rapidly than adults was known a century ago. This is still the case today. However, the profound increase in the severity of Type 2 hypothyroidism and environmental illnesses means more youngsters have difficulty tolerating thyroid hormones. Infants may only require one-quarter grain. Children may use one-half to one and one-half grains. A few of my early teenage patients need as much as three grains, especially if they are large people. The basal temperature and heart rate are critical factors for monitoring dosages in the young. Their temperatures almost always normalize with proper thyroid and iodine treatment. Many adults' basal temperatures remain below normal despite proper treatment. This is problably due to their increased burden of environmental toxins and mitochondrial defects.

Dr. Barnes advocated having patients monitor their basal temperatures on a monthly basis until the proper dosage was attained. His research demonstrated that as long as the patients' basal temperature remained at or below 98.2 °F, the patients would not suffer any ill effects. Increased heart rate, nervousness, tremor, increased problems sleeping, weight loss, excessive sweating, and elevated basal temperature are all signs of too much thyroid hormone. **If a basal temperature rose above 98.2 °F, an immediate reduction in the dosage was indicated**.

Many of my pain patients ran very low temperatures. Two patients reported 93 °F. Despite large dosages of up to four grains of desiccated thyroid, their temperatures increased but failed to reach the normal range. Adding more thyroid frequently caused side effects. However, the vast majority of patients' symptoms improved despite their continued low temperatures.

It was reassuring to hear Dr. Barnes speak on the research tapes that are available through his foundation. He stated that he was unable to attain temperatures in the normal range with many of his patients. Despite persistent lower than normal basal temperatures, patients' symptoms vastly improved and chronic illnesses were rare in those he cared for.

The hormone disrupting chemicals and other environmentally related illnesses all share the blame for the persistence of low basal temperatures and metabolism despite maximal thyroid hormone replacement. One of the giants in the field of environmental medicine is William Rea M.D. He has reported normalization of low basal temperatures and hypothyroid-like symptoms after the patients have undergone detoxification without utilizing thyroid hormones. More about Dr. Rea's work and environmental medicine will be discussed in Chapter 12.

Adequate supplementation of iodine and iodide are necessary for proper thyroid and steroid hormone function. **Many patients may not tolerate or respond to desiccated thyroid unless relatively large dosages of iodine/iodide are administered.** Too much iodine can be lethal and must be used judiciously (please consult your physician).[99]

Rats deprived of either iron or selenium will develop hypo-thyroidism. Both are critical for the utilization of thyroid hormones. The Barnes Foundation recommends an iron (ferritin) level over 100 ng/ml. Ferritin levels over 130 are advised for menstruating women. Most of my female patients have ferritin levels far below those recommended by the Barnes Foundation. Adult males are much less apt to be deficient. Patients may not respond well to, or may require a higher dosage of, desiccated thyroid until their iron levels are raised. Ferrous glycine is a type of iron that is chelated (chemically joined) with glycine, an amino acid. Patients tolerate this form of iron much better than other forms, and it is available commercially. A number of patients reported recurrences of hypothyroid symptoms if they missed a few days of iron replacement. Too much iron in the blood can cause serious problems; therefore, a doctor needs to monitor the dosage.

Selenium is recommended for all my patients suffering hypothyroidism, between 200 mcg and 400 mcg per day. Selenium deficiencies are common among our populace. A group of selenium-containing enzymes has been shown necessary for proper conversion and metabolism of thyroid.[73] Too much selenium, however, can also cause problems.

The vast majority of my patients have a milieu of expensive prescriptions except for the one they need the most, desiccated thyroid. If hypothyroidism and environmental illnesses were properly treated, most medications consumed by our chronically ill society would no longer be necessary.

Chapter 10
Why Patients Do Not Tolerate Desiccated
Thyroid and Mild Adrenal Deficiencies

The day after discovering the Barnes Foundation in the spring of 1999, I telephoned its director. My first question was, "Why don't some of my hypothyroid patients tolerate even the smallest dosages of thyroid hormones?" The health of many of my patients, friends, and family depended upon the answer. Their answer was, "They are adrenally insufficient." In order for thyroid medication to raise a person's metabolism, their adrenal glands must be able to function adequately. Without the necessary adrenal hormones, such as cortisol, patients either do not tolerate or are unable to properly convert the main thyroid hormone (T4) into the much more physiologically active form (T3).

In many patients, the problem turned out to be much more complicated than just adrenal deficiencies. Other complicating factors include iodine and magnesium deficiencies, stomach and intestinal problems such as Candidiasis, food allergies, and the environmental poisons such as mercury that interfere with hundreds of biochemical reactions and contaminate us all (see Chapter 12).

Another great pioneer who remains largely unrecognized in the field of endocrinology was William Jefferies M.D. The Barnes Foundation promotes his book entitled, *Safe Uses of Cortisol*. Dr. Jefferies devoted his career to treating patients as well as doing research. His study of how adrenal hormones function began in the 1950s, very shortly after scientists first isolated the adrenal steroids.[63]

Historically, most doctors have been taught that the adrenal glands either work well or not at all. Dr. Jefferies described the concept of mild adrenal deficiency in detail in 1981 when the first edition of his book was published. Dr. Barnes also addressed the topic of mild adrenal insufficiency in his chapter devoted to the treatment of arthritis.[4]

Dr. Jefferies addressed topics of allergic disorders, autoimmune disorders, chronic fatigue, infertility, viral infections such as colds, flu, mononucleosis, shingles, as well as other problems that may result from or be partially attributable to the adrenal glands.

Additional symptoms of adrenal deficiency include feeling hot all the time, palpitations, low blood pressure (systolic of 100 or less), very slender build, dizziness (especially on standing up quickly), severe allergies, anxiety and feelings of impending doom, hypoglycemia, arthritis, weakness, and fatigue after exercise. There is much overlap between the symptoms resulting from hypothyroidism and adrenal insufficiency. Dr. Jefferies explains why proper thyroid function may not be attained without an assist from the adrenal glands.

One important class of adrenal steroids is called "gluco-corticoids." The prime function of the glucocorticoids is to stimulate the formation of glucose, the body's chief source of energy. The major glucocorticoid produced by our adrenals is cortisol, also called "hydrocortisone". Without glucocorticoids, we would die within several days. They are essential for life as well as the maintenance of a long list of tasks required for health and well-being.

Dr. Jefferies' book is entitled *Safe Uses of Cortisol* for a reason. Different forms of cortisol were made available for human trials in 1948. Unfortunately, large dosages were used that exceeded the normal amounts that circulate in our blood. The excessive dosages initially used to medicate patients gave rise to terrible side effects including osteoporosis and spontaneous fractures, fluid retention, thin skin with hemorrhages and bruising, stomach ulcers, decreased immunity to infections, as well as other alarming problems. The stigmata associated with these initial reports continue to linger in medical textbooks even today. Doctors are still taught to use these steroids such as prednisone, a glucocorticoid, as a last resort and with caution. In the U.S., only an extremely small number of doctors familiar with Dr. Jefferies' work and the Barnes Foundation have ever used low-dose cortisol or prednisone to treat mild adrenal insufficiency.

Prednisone is a synthetic glucocorticoid derived from cortisone and has similar effects. Prednisone remains one of the only medications found effective against a number of chronic illnesses. Doctors routinely place patients on prednisone for problems such as asthma, lupus, rheumatoid arthritis, and other chronic illnesses. Yet, it is almost unheard of for doctors to check the patients' adrenal function prior to beginning treatment. Unfortunately, even if performed, the "standard" adrenal tests do not identify most cases of mild adrenal insufficiency.

Dr. Jefferies realized the "standard" tests for adrenal deficiency failed to detect the majority of mild cases. The "normal" values on standard adrenal tests utilized by major universities and laboratories are in stark contrast with those he advocated. Dr. Jefferies also stated that many patients may test "within the normal range" on his scale and yet require small dosages of adrenal hormones to restore their health. Most patients with mild adrenal deficiencies often require only a very small dosage of cortisol, such as two and one-half milligrams, two or three times a day, to remain healthy. A few may need a total of 20 to 30 milligrams per day.

Dr. Barnes used the minimum amount of adrenal steroids such as prednisone or cortisol that would allow his patients to either tolerate or respond to desiccated thyroid.

A study published in 1950 by Drs. George W. Thorn and S. Richardson Hill from Harvard reviewed the closely intertwined, physiological relationship between adrenal steroids and thyroid function. Their study revealed that supra-physiological dosages of adrenal steroids greatly inhibited thyroid function. "Physiological dosage" is the normal dosage present in the body. The authors stated, "The second phase of adrenal steroid influence on thyroid function is an inhibitory one in which all aspects of thyroid function are depressed."[66] Here was the reason why the early use of prednisone-like drugs had resulted in severe osteoporosis and suppressed immune function, because the doctors had overdosed their patients without knowing that too much cortisol would turn off normal thyroid function.

Nearly all of the problems associated with the use of physiological dosages of glucocorticoids are avoided when sufficient dosages of desiccated thyroid are administered. Drs. Jefferies, Barnes, and Hertoghe have all published studies clearly showing beneficial results from physiological dosages of glucocorticoids given to patients with mild adrenal insufficiency and adequate desiccated thyroid. A thorough search of the medical literature revealed no studies showing adverse effects.

In the early twentieth century, many doctors recognized that the vast majority of arthritic patients suffered hypothyroidism. Thyroid extract was the preferred treatment for all forms of arthritis and rheumatism.[2,32,97] Dr. Barnes recognized the majority of arthritic patients also suffered from mild adrenal deficiency. After finding the 1950 study by Thorn and Hill, Dr. Barnes treated hundreds of arthritic patients by giving them physiological dosages of glucocorticoids combined with desiccated thyroid. He noted an absence of ill effects and a remarkable improvement in their symptoms.[4,10]

Dr. Barnes advocated beginning with thyroid hormones and adding the adrenal hormones later, unless the patient was unable to tolerate thyroid medication. He did not like the idea of potentially suppressing thyroid function by starting with adrenal hormones.

A growing number of doctors currently start patients on thyroid treatment by using adrenal hormones initially and adding thyroid replacement four to seven days later. Prior to the last two years, I would start thyroid within one or two days of beginning low dose adrenal steroids, if necessary. I now start with iodine/iodide from one to four weeks to allow the adrenals to regain normal function and then begin one-quarter grain of thyroid in most patients with mild adrenal deficiency. The liberal usage of iodine and iodide in my practice has markedly decreased my patients' requirement for adrenal steroids. The combination of desiccated thyroid along with ample iodine/iodide appears to be a potent remedy for mild adrenal deficiencies.

My preferred form of iodine/iodide is Lugol's Strong Iodine Solution. I have a compounding pharmacy dispense it in one ounce (29.5 cc) dropper bottles. Patients begin with one drop that they rub into their skin and increase one drop every four or five days. Most adults require four drops a day (25mg) for optimal benefits. Children need less. Refer to Dr. Brownstein's book for more details.[99]

In my opinion, it appears most patients who require adrenal steroids, despite adequate iodine/iodide replacement, have root canal teeth and/or chronic infections of the jaws. These chronic dental infections are sources of severe stress on the body that results in adrenal deficiency and impaired immunity. Remediation of these infections and other chronic infections in my patients has resulted in the resolution of most of their adrenal deficiencies.[106]

Iodine receptors are present in every one of our trillions of cells. Hormone producing tissues are particularly dependent upon normal levels of iodine to function properly. For optimal health, Americans require many times the amount of iodine/iodide we receive from our diet and iodized salt. David Brownstein M.D. has compelling research about iodine in his book, *Iodine: Why You Need It, Why You Can't Live Without It*.[99] Research reveals that there are crucial iodine receptors in all the endocrine glands. Iodine is in a class of molecules called halides and is an essential element. Other halides include chlorine, bromine, and fluorine, which are ubiquitous toxins in our water and food. Dr. Brownstein's research shows how these toxic halides are displaced from the iodine receptors when patients take adequate amounts of iodine. He also presents evidence that shows iodine may help prevent autoimmune illnesses, prostate, and breast cancer.[99] (www.drbrownstein.com)

A must read book is *Breast Cancer and Iodine* by David Derry M.D., Ph.D. The research in his book also reveals the vital importance of iodine for optimal health and the prevention of many cancers. [107] A listing of Dr. Derry's proposed functions of iodine are found on the next page.

Dr. Derry's Proposed Functions of Iodine

1. Used to make thyroid hormone in thyroid gland.
2. Main body surveillance mechanism for abnormal cells in body.
3. Triggers Apoptosis (program death of cells) in normal cells and abnormal cells.
4. Detoxifies chemicals.
5. Reacts with tyrosine and histidine to inactivate enzymes and denature protein.
6. Antiseptic to bacteria, algae, fungi, viruses and protozoa.
7. Detoxifies biological toxins food poisoning, snake venoms, etc.
8. Anti-allergic process. Makes external proteins non-allergic.
9. Anti-autoimmune mechanism by making intracellular proteins spilled into blood non-allergic.
10. Protection of double bonds in lipids for delivery to cardiovascular system and synaptic membranes in brain and retina.
11. Fetal source of apoptitic mechanisms during development in fetus and breast-fed children.
12. Protection from apoptotic diseases such as leukemia.
13. Possible initial source of thyroxine in early fetal development.
14. Antiseptic activity in stomach against heliobacter pylori. [107]
15. Iodine causes regeneration of human scars to normal skin. [108,109]

Another important element in our diets that can interfere with a patients' ability to have normal thyroid function is magnesium. *The Scientific Basis for Environmental Medicine Techniques,* authored by Sherry Rogers M.D., includes a discussion of the diagnosis and treatment of magnesium deficiency. Magnesium is integral to the activity and function of enzymes vital to our health. Magnesium deficiency can cause irritability of the muscles, including the heart, and the nervous system. Without adequate magnesium, thyroid hormones are more likely to cause rapid or irregular heartbeats. Many patients require 600 to 1,000 milligrams of high quality magnesium daily until their deficiency resolves. A few patients with more severe gastrointestinal or kidney problems only respond to magnesium oil or intravenous magnesium therapy. These patients often suffer diarrhea from taking oral magnesium preparations. The standard blood test for magnesium does not reflect cellular levels of the element. Therefore, this test is not accurate.

Some environmentally ill patients are often sensitive to or intolerant of both adrenal and thyroid hormones. As previously mentioned, one of the pioneers in chemical sensitivities is William Rea M.D. Dr. Rea published studies documenting resolution of adrenal deficiencies after treatment for environmental illnesses. I went to study at his treatment center in Dallas, Texas. During our first meeting, I expressed frustration regarding my inability to treat many environmentally ill patients with hormones. "They are too toxic, aren't they?" he responded with a wry smile. I nodded in agreement. Many chronically ill patients require treatment for their environmental illnesses and toxicity before beginning thyroid hormone treatment. Additionally, chronic exposure to mold in the home or at work is a frequent finding among many of my sick patients who do not tolerate desiccated thyroid hormones.[41]

A 40 year-old female patient with fatigue, cold intolerance, dry skin and hair, irregular menses, and chronic pain was intolerant of the smallest thyroid dosage. Her heart rate shot up, and she developed tremors. Testing showed her mercury level to be over 15 times greater than normal. After treatment to lower her mercury, she was able to tolerate three grains of thyroid and her symptoms greatly improved.

I continue to refine the delicate balancing act of increasing thyroid and adrenal hormones simultaneously. Every patient is different and each requires special attention. Patients with severe chronic pain are frequently difficult to balance hormonally. The blame probably lies with their environmental toxins and illnesses. A patient may require very small dosages of cortisol and thyroid made by formulating pharmacies, because the commercially available preparations are too strong. Occasionally, patients are allergic to the fillers or additives in pills such as cornstarch contained in commercial thyroid and cortisol. A very gradual increase in their in their hormone replacement over a period of years may be required before complete restoration of health occurs.

Patients who require cortisol for adrenal deficiency must have a home blood pressure monitor or I will not participate in their care. Too much or too little cortisol frequently affects patients' blood pressure. If they have problems with their medication, they are instructed to take their blood pressure and heart rate before taking a dosage of cortisol. Next, they report their blood pressure and heart rate an hour and a half to two hours later. Cortisol works fast. If their blood pressure normalizes and other adrenal symptoms respond favorably, they obviously needed the increased dose of cortisol. If the opposite occurs, they may be taking too much cortisol and the dose may need to be lowered. **If the patient is on too much thyroid (or is intolerant), their heart rate usually increases, often without appreciable blood pressure changes.**

The Barnes Foundation, the Drs. Hertoghe, and I recommend prednisolone as an alternative to cortisol. Prednisolone is another glucocorticoid that is similar to prednisone. Prednisolone need only be taken once a day, where cortisol is taken one to four times a day. Prednisolone is less likely to cause the fluid retention that occasionally results from taking cortisol. Children and teenagers almost invariably prefer the single daily dosage.

Case Study

A 70 year old female, taking 4 grains (240 mg) of Amour thyroid since age 17 presents herself to my clinic. Her physician had died. Her new university endocrinologist cut her dosage to 2 grains (120 mg) because her TSH was less than 0.01 (i.e. suppressed). Within 3 months she had a 30 pound weigh gain, was unable to balance her checkbook, could not articulate her thoughts and experienced severe fatigue.

A. DEXA scan (bone density test): T-score minus 1.1, 95% aged matched Z-score minus 0.4. (a normal reading).

B. Stress test (heart): 115% of age predicted maximum. Heart rate 173 at peak exercise, ejection fraction 75% with no evidence of significant ischemia (no restricted blood flow). (a normal reading).

C. All symptoms resolved shortly after she resumed 4 grains of thyroid.

This case illustrates that long-term suppression of the TSH does not result in the predicted osteoporosis or heart problems current dogma about TSH suggests. My patient's bone density (DEXA scan) and heart tests were basically normal.

Chapter 11
Female and Male Hormonal
Relationships to Thyroid Hormone
And the Women's Health Initiative

The Shorr Stain: The Missing Link in the Evaluation
And Treatment of Estrogen Deficiency

Proper function of thyroid hormones allows each cell to perform normally. The mitochondria discussion in Chapter 6 describes their profound influence on endocrine glands. Further evidence supporting the connection between hypothyroidism, other hormone problems, and environmental toxins is discussed in Chapter 12.

Hypothyroidism often results in impotence in men and decreased libido in both sexes. Deficiencies of testosterone, low sperm counts, and testicular atrophy are possible. Once firmly entrenched, these problems may not resolve with thyroid hormone treatment alone. I prescribe testosterone for a large number of my patients, women as well as men. Low adrenal output and ovarian dysfunction have long been associated with low thyroid function. More severe problems involving multiple hormone disorders have developed and are rearing their ugly heads at a much younger age.

Drs. Sonkin and Cohen published a treatise in 1969 entitled, *Treatment of the Menopause*. In it they stated, "The menopause has been of special interest in the Endocrine Clinic of the New York Hospital–Cornell Medical Center since 1934, when Dr. Ephraim Shorr and Dr. George Papanicolaou reported on the action of estrogens in ovarian-insufficient women, and the measurement of hormone response by examination of specially stained vaginal smears." Clinical applications for evaluating individual estrogen levels in women by the vaginal smear were first published in a 1945 medical journal. Dr. Sonkin correctly noted the bibliography in the journal article by Drs. Shorr and Papanicolaou contained the names of "the giants in the fields of endocrinology and cytology."

Cytology is the study of cells, their origin, structure, functions, and pathology.[74,75] The "Shorr stain" proved invaluable in the treatment of female hormone disorders. Dr. Papanicolaou is also renowned for introducing the "PAP" smear.

Dr. Sonkin taught me how to check women's estrogen levels by utilizing the Shorr stain. The stain allows doctors to tell if a woman's ovaries are producing the proper amount of estrogen during different times in the menstrual cycle. The estrogen levels peak during ovulation. This is called the "estrus". Estrus occurs at midcycle, prior to the onset of progesterone production. At the peak of estrus, the vaginal cells mature and take on a characteristic appearance, which can be seen by swabbing the vagina and looking at the cells under a microscope after using the Shorr stain.[74]

Estrogen requirements vary considerably among women. Modern blood tests for estrogen levels only show the average amount of hormone for large female populations of similar age and menstrual status. Each individual's precise requirement may only be revealed by the Shorr stain. The following graph is taken from the original research paper published by Drs. Shorr and Papanicolaou. Notice the elongated tail of the graph to the right of the large bell curve. The women represented by this portion need a much higher blood level of estrogen than the "average" to function normally.

Range of Dosage Required for Estrus in Human Females

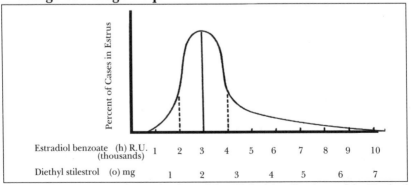

Source: Shorr, E. 1945. An Evaluation of the Clinical Applications of the Vaginal Smear Method. *Journal of the Mount Sinai Hospital* May-June; XII(1):667-688. Reprinted with permission.

During the tenure of Drs. Papanicolaou and Shorr, the dosages of estrogen given at the New York Hospital–Cornell Medical Center Endocrine Clinics ranged from 0.3 mg to 10 mg of Premarin® (the only type of oral estrogen available at the time). Drs. Cohen and Sonkin stated, "An occasional patient proves both subjectively and biologically resistant to the effects of oral hormone therapy confirmed by lack of cellular development in the vaginal smear. Such patients usually respond to parenteral [intramuscular injections] estrogens in dosages as high as 20 to 40 mg of estradiol valerate every 7 to 10 days." Dosages this large are unfathomable (excessive) among our modern endocrinologists. (The "standard" dosage of Premarin® has remained 0.625 mg.) These historical giants in the field of endocrinology utilized the stain until the end of their careers. The Shorr stain proved invaluable for the correct diagnosis and treatment of estrogen disorders in women of all ages. Relief from menopausal symptoms coincided with maturation of their vaginal cells determined by the Shorr stain, reflecting adequate estrogen replacement. Decades of research on estrogen's effects and the menopause by the world's preeminent doctors and institutions has long been forgotten.

Menopausal symptoms may include hot flushes, drenching sweats, tingling of the extremities, muscle pain, headaches, irritability, apathy, loss of capability, vertigo, depression, vaginitis, and recurrent urinary tract infections. The prognosis for symptomatic relief is much better if estrogen is given sooner rather than later in suffering women.[75]

Dr. Sonkin believed estrogens used properly (as determined by the Shorr stain), combined with thyroid therapy when indicated, might be protective against breast cancer. Dr. Sonkin related to me that breast cancer in his patients was quite rare.

The Women's Health Initiative (WHI) was a very large-scale study of both the beneficial and adverse effects of hormone replacement for menopausal women.[104] The study purportedly showed a very slight increase risk of heart attack, stroke, and breast cancer for women using Premarin. As a result, millions of women around the world either chose or were forced by their doctors to stop their hormone replacement therapy (HRT). M.E. Ted Quigley M.D., a gynecologist, spent years of his spare time examining the WHI data. He uncovered profound flaws in the design of the study.

Like Dr. Sonkin, Dr. Quigley had seen the great benefits women enjoyed from using HRT. He was not aware of any cases of breast cancer in his patients receiving HRT during 25 years of clinical practice.

In clinical practice, women are begun on HRT around the time of their menopause, typically in their 40s and 50s. Prior research studies have shown the greatest benefits such as decreased coronary artery disease were obtained when HRT was begun within several years of menopause.

Three age groups of women (161,808) were enrolled in the WHI. They were ages 50-59, 60-69, and 70-79. Only 6% of these women were on HRT when the study began and 75% had never taken hormones. The women were said to have been healthy. However, 36% were taking high blood pressure medicine, 13% were on cholesterol lowering drugs, and 6% had coronary vascular disease.[105]

One portion of the WHI study was devoted to women (11,000) who had prior hysterectomies. The hysterectomized women were divided into groups receiving: A) Premarin (estrogen), B) Premarin plus Provera (progestin), and C) placebo (no drug). The 50-59 year-old women taking Premarin were compared to the women taking placebo. There was a 44% reduction in heart attacks, a 28% reduction in invasive breast cancer, a 27% reduction in deaths, and no increased risk of stroke. The benefits of taking estrogen decreased in the older age groups.

In the 50-59 year old group of women taking Premarin plus Provera (versus placebo), there was a 26% increase in heart attacks and a 20% increase in breast cancer.

Dr. Quigley's conclusions regarding WHI were that unhealthy, older, postmenopausal women who delayed initiation of HRT for many years after menopause had a small increased risk of heart attack, breast cancer, or stroke that was not statistically significant. Synthetic progestins appear to increase the risk of coronary artery disease, invasive breast cancer, stroke, and deep venous thrombosis (blood clots in legs).

Obviously, there appears to be significant benefits associated with using estrogen around the time of menopause. I highly recommend doctors and patients read Dr. Quigley's soon to be released book, *MeNoPause: Awaken & Empower YourSelf*.[103]

Recent research has shown many more beneficial effects and far fewer side effects when "natural" human bio-identical hormones are used. Our cell's hormone receptors are structured like a lock and key to fit individual hormones. Alterations in these crucial hormones often result in untoward side effects. Hormones identical to those produced in our bodies are readily available from formulating pharmacies. Pharmaceutical companies cannot patent the natural hormones and do not promote their research. Hence, pharmacologically produced synthetic hormones are generally prescribed for the average patient.[76,77]

With few exceptions, my premenopausal patients suffering from pain and hypothyroidism also had evidence of estrogen deficiency (ovarian dysfunction) on their Shorr stains. Two of those suffering chronic musculoskeletal pain and estrogen deficiency were in their 20s. One of the two developed endometriosis. Unfortunately, I had not yet realized the pervasiveness of hypothyroidism, nor had I learned to use iodine/iodide.

There is a growing body of literature attributing "estrogen dominance" to a large number of female maladies. Weight gain, irregular and heavy periods, PMS, depression, migraines, blood clotting problems, fibroids, ovarian cysts, endometriosis, and breast cancer are the main symptoms blamed on the estrogen dominance theory. These symptoms are all included on the list for hypothyroidism and iodine deficiencies.

Estrogen dominance is in essence a progesterone deficiency. The mainstay of treatment for estrogen dominance is transdermal, bio-identical progesterone cream. Headaches, insomnia, decreased libido, mood swings, and fluid retention are some of the symptoms that often respond very well to natural progesterone. *What Your Doctor May Not Tell You About Premenopause* by John R. Lee M.D. is an excellent book about the benefits of bio-identical progesterone.

The ovaries concentrate large amounts of iodine, second only to the thyroid gland. Iodine and iodide are critical components for all of our hormone producing tissues. The proper balance of estrogens may not be attained without adequate supplementation of these elements.[99]

Andropause
The male equivalent of menopause is termed "andropause". Diminished libido and potency, fatigue, loss of muscle mass and endurance, depression, a lack of drive or assertiveness, and

increased perspiration are possible symptoms from declining levels of testosterone. Testosterone replacement usually reverses the loss of muscle mass associated with aging. The heart muscle also benefits. Low levels of testosterone, as well as other endocrine dysfunction, such as hypothyroidism must be addressed to restore the affected men's health. Treatment of environmentally related illnesses and toxicities is often necessary to optimize outcomes.[40,41,75,78]

Malcomb Carruthers M.D., author of *The Testosterone Revolution*, is the director of the largest study of male andropause. The Website for this ongoing study based in London is: www.andropause.org.uk

Methyltestosterone, a form of synthetic testosterone, was banned in Europe many years ago, due to potential liver toxicity. Dr. Carruthers was shocked when I informed him that it continues to be prescribed in America. Testosterone cream, identical to human testosterone, is less expensive, much safer, more effective, and has been available from compounding pharmacies for years in America. An inexpensive, bio-identical oral testosterone named Andriol® is available throughout Europe and Canada, but is curiously unavailable in America.

Proper treatment with human bio-identical testosterone has proven safe in Dr. Carruther's large study group. High levels of human testosterone do not increase the incidence of prostate cancer. In fact, the treatment group has a lower incidence than men in the general population.

A few of our teaching institutions have established alternative medicine departments; however, they are still the exception rather than the rule. One doctor with whom I visited resigned her position at a university, because it had taken as long as three years to receive approval for her alternative treatment protocols.

Treating the underlying causes of a chronic disease is much more efficacious than treating the resultant symptoms. Prevention is the ultimate goal.

The International College of Integrative Medicine (www.icimed.com), The American College for Advancement in Medicine (www.acam.org), and American Holistic Medical Association (www.holisticmedicine.org) are possible sources of help.

Chapter 12
Environmental Toxins = Hormonal Havoc

Readers note: This chapter includes many valuable tables and charts that disrupted the flow of the chapter when embedded in the text. Therefore, they have been added to the end of the chapter and referenced by table number.

Introduction

Environmental toxins are now commonplace. There is no escaping exposure to industrial wastes, pesticides, and other pollutants including toxic chemicals. Toxic chemicals are pervasive in our food, water, and air. About 70,000 new synthetic chemicals were introduced into our environment during the twentieth century. Three-quarters of the 20 most toxic chemical pollutants are known to be poisonous to our nervous systems. The list of synthetic chemicals that interfere with thyroid and other hormone functions is rapidly expanding. **Eighty percent of these new chemicals have never been screened for their effects on human health.**

In the twenty-first century, everyone (including newborn children) is encumbered with scores of chemical toxins no matter how remote their place of origin. From the most isolated parts of Alaska and China, to the farthest points of civilization north and south, we are all affected. I will highlight several predominant classes of pollutants with an emphasis on those known to adversely affect thyroid metabolism.

Toxins may begin to exact their toll on a person prior to conception. The health of an infant can be jeopardized by chemically induced genetic damage to the father's sperm or mother's egg. Medical studies have shown that men and women frequently exposed to pesticides in their work exhibit a number of such genetic mutations.[41]

Food Contamination

Over one billion tons of pesticides are used in the United States every year. The top ten pesticides used are all herbicides. These usually find their way into our food and water supplies. An EPA survey shows that all commercially grown foods in America have pesticides in them. Table 12.1 reveals common chemical contaminants found in commercially produced food are almost absent in organically grown food.[67]

See Table 12.1 at end of chapter

Animals crowded into feedlots are given antibiotics and treated with pesticides. These animals are also dependent upon commercially produced foods treated with insecticides and herbicides. All of these toxins accumulate in their body tissues and are readily passed on to consumers. Many of these pesticides, insecticides, and herbicides interfere with thyroid metabolism.[35,67]

Bad things often happen to our food supply during preparation, storage, and transportation. Food additives include preservatives, flavorings, colorings, and dyes. Bleaching foods like French fries with sulfuric acid and chlorines can add to their toxic burden. Fungicides and fumigants are sprayed directly on perishables to delay spoiling and protect them from insects. Containers may be oiled and treated with pesticides, acrylics, or other toxic substances that leach into the foods. Synthetic chemicals that make plastic flexible are called "phthalates". These and other toxins leach out of the plastic to contaminate the food or drink they are supposed to protect. A section is devoted to phthalates later in this chapter. Many of these contaminants adversely affect thyroid metabolism and interfere with estrogen and testosterone. Table 12.2 highlights common sources of food contamination during transportation, storage, and preparation.[67]

See Table 12.2 at end of chapter

Water Pollution

Numerous chemicals and other toxins pollute our drinking and bathing water. Chlorinated city water contains 100 to 10,000 times as many synthetic compounds as natural spring water. It is estimated that we absorb several times more of these pollutants from bathing than from drinking. Most toxins are fat soluble and easily absorbed directly through our skin or the membranes that line our lungs and gut. Trihalomethanes are by-products from the chlorination process that kill germs and microorganisms. Trihalomethanes are toxic to humans. Chlorine combines with organic material to form these and other toxic by-products. Many of these toxic chemicals are known to disrupt thyroid metabolism and cause cancer.

Benzene derivatives and similar compounds were analyzed in the drinking water derived from the Mississippi River. In Minneapolis, near the river's source, there were only 14.5 parts per billion (ppb) trihalomethanes. The number had risen to 108 ppb in East St. Louis (half way through its course). New Orleans' drinking water contained 156 ppb just before it reached the Gulf of Mexico. The EPA set 100 ppb as the safe drinking water standard. Other pollutants such as arsenic, mercury, PCBs, and dioxins disrupt thyroid metabolism. These are also found in drinking water supplies. Table 12.3 illustrates the correlation of contaminants found in drinking water and those found in the blood from ailing patients at the Environmental Health Center in Dallas (EHCD).[67] Many of the contaminants are common to both.

See Table 12.3 at end of chapter

Drinking water that contains fluoride may be a major contributor to Type 2 hypothyroidism. Fluoride has been proven to destroy thyroid gland tissue in dosages simular to those found in our water. For more information see www.fluoridealert.org and www.slweb.org

Air Pollution

Most air pollution easily passes through our bodies' protective barriers, particularly the lungs. Adults inhale close to three metric tons of air each year (4.3 liters per minute). Hence, minute amounts of pollutants found in the atmosphere can accumulate in our bodies over time. As industrialization during the twentieth century flourished, so, too, did toxic emissions.

Emissions from one part of the world often ride the trade winds to other countries and continents to have far reaching consequences. Pesticides sprayed to control grasshoppers in Africa were detected five days later in Florida. Factory emissions of nitrous oxides and sulfur dioxides end up as acid rain in Canada up to 2,000 miles from their American source. Nuclear fallout from the 1987 Chernobyl explosion traversed the circumference of our earth, and radioactive fallout was distributed globally from extensive Soviet and American nuclear bomb testing in the 1950s and 1960s. The fallout no doubt contributed to the genetic defects affecting thyroid metabolism. The general circulation of air currents around our earth is due to the forces resulting from the earth's rotation, called the "Coriolis Effect". Circulation patterns are represented in Table 12.4.[67]

See Table 12.4 at end of chapter

In 1989, the EPA estimated the amount of toxic air chemicals released by American industry. Almost 2.5 billion pounds were released by industries. These tables do not include tens of millions of cars or other private and natural sources such as volcanoes and forest fires. The rest of the rapidly industrializing world's contributions are also not included. Sources of pollutants released by industries are listed in Table 12.5.

See Table 12.5 at end of chapter

Noted Toxic Effects of Pollution on Thyroid Metabolism

> The most disturbing aspect of chemical toxins may be their ability to disrupt the function of thyroid hormones. Thyroid metabolism is one of the most frequent targets of synthetic chemicals.

Nothing is safe from environmental toxins, not even the developing human fetus. Chemical and environmental toxins cross the placenta of every expectant mother to reach her unborn fetus. Drugs and alcohol, heavy metals like lead and mercury, and toxic chemicals such as the pesticides that contaminate our food and water are all able to infiltrate the placenta.

The developing fetus is extraordinarily sensitive to the toxins that all of us now harbor. Many common offenders can damage DNA or alter genes and genetic expression. The fetus' ability to detoxify poisons is lacking. The kidneys, liver, and lungs are the primary organs responsible for detoxification and are non-functional during the crucial early stages of gestation.

The majority of toxic chemicals are deposited and stored in our fat. Many of the most widely studied and ubiquitous toxins are quite persistent and remain in our bodies for many years or decades. With continued daily exposure to even minute amounts of this pollutant milieu, our "total load" of toxins gradually increases.

Part of a mother's milk to nurse her babies is derived from her fat stores. The milk is rich in fat as well as chemical toxins she has spent her lifetime accumulating. Each successive generation is burdened with increasingly larger "total toxic loads." A growing body of evidence reveals the insidious effects upon every aspect of our being that may result from this exposure.

Breast-feeding remains far superior to infant formula despite concerns about toxins. Most infant formulas are derived from soybeans. Twenty-first century soybeans grown in America are almost all "genetically engineered". This allows the plants to be more resistant to the effects of pesticides. Therefore, more pesticides are used to ensure larger crop yields. Soybeans are one of the most common foods known to cause food allergies. Babies that are repeatedly fed soy formulas are likely to develop significant food allergy problems.

A diet rich in soy also inhibits thyroid metabolism. A recent study published in the *Alternative Medicine Review* involved 37 adults who ate a diet high in soy for three months. Almost half of the subjects developed hypothyroid symptoms including malaise, constipation, sleepiness, and goiters. These symptoms resolved one month after stopping the diet.[79]

Soy products are also used to treat symptoms of menopause. Soy has a high content of plant estrogens called "phytoestrogens". Infants fed soy had concentrations of phytoestrogens 13,000 to

22,000 greater than their concentration of natural estrogens. These soy estrogens may interfere with the infants' own estrogen and testosterone.[79]

Thyroid hormones orchestrate the development of our brain. These hormones stimulate the unborn fetus' genes to produce brain cells. Thyroid influences the migration and branching of the nerves to their proper locations while making the correct interconnections. They stimulate formation of the insulation sheath called myelin that protects the nerves from short-circuiting while communicating messages to different parts of the brain.[91]

A research article published in 2002 by Dr. Kembra Howdeshell detailed the great importance of the thyroid hormones' influence on the development of the brain. A review of the studies documenting synthetic chemical interference with thyroid metabolism and brain development was also presented in the same article. In it she stated, "Indeed, synthetic chemicals can disrupt nearly every step in the production and metabolism of thyroid hormone." She continued, "The ability of man-made chemicals to disrupt the thyroid system strongly suggests the possibility of chemical perturbation of thyroid-sensitive brain development." A list of synthetic chemicals that interfere with thyroid metabolism from this research paper appears in Appendix B.[80]

The problem is pervasive. The list of synthetic chemicals with thyroid disruption properties published in 1998 by Dr. Françoise Brucker-Davis, a research scientist from the World Wildlife Fund, only begins to elucidate its magnitude.[81]

See Table 12.6 at end of chapter

The best research scientists in the world, including Dr. Brucker-Davis, have heavily relied upon thyroid blood tests to determine the impact of toxins on thyroid function. As discussed in Chapter 7, these blood tests rarely detect Type 2 hypothyroidism. Therefore, there is little doubt that the deleterious effects on thyroid metabolism are much more profound than indicated by recent research. Powerful support for these concepts is demonstrated by studies on affected patients. Dr. Rea reports many patients who exhibited classical symptoms of hypothyroidism returned to health after they underwent detoxification and treatment for their environmental illnesses. They did not require thyroid supplements.

Animal studies are particularly useful when studying hormones. For example, all vertebrates have very similar steroid hormone metabolism. Steroids (hormones) are all derived from cholesterol and include testosterone, estrogen, and progesterone. Both male and female vertebrates require all three of these hormones for health. Males require higher levels of testosterone and less estrogen and progesterone than females. Thyroid hormones are also uniformly preserved among the vertebrates.

The Toxic Chemicals Known To Affect Thyroid Function

PCBs

PCBs (polychlorinated biphenyls) were used as nonflammable coolant fluids in capacitors and electrical transformers. First synthesized in 1929, PCBs are extremely stable compounds and have proven to be extraordinarily useful in the electrification and industrialization of Western Civilization. Over 200 variations of these molecules were widely used as lubricants, hydraulic fluids, inks, paints, varnishes, adhesives, pesticides, and to make wood and rubber nonflammable. During the 1960s, the PCB buildup in air, fresh water, soil, oceans, birds, fish, and mammals became apparent. PCBs have now been shown to inhibit thyroid function.

In 1977, the production of PCBs was banned in America. The rest of the world (such as the Soviet Union in 1990), eventually followed. The ban did not address existing PCBs that continued to leach from old capacitors, transformers, and a multitude of other sources. Some of the most persistent PCBs are only broken down by ultraviolet B radiation from the sun. The pervasive presence of PCBs and many similar toxins bodes ill for future generations of animal life on our planet.

PCBs and other persistent toxins are biomagnified. Their concentration in water may be miniscule. However, they begin to accumulate in the fatty tissues of organisms low in the food chain. As each successive ladder in the chain is climbed, and larger animals consume smaller ones, an exponential increase in the persistent agent occurs. Animals at the top of the food chain may harbor many million times the pollutant's concentration in water or sediments.

The following illustration is from *Our Stolen Future*.[82] The book's authors are responsible for much of the pioneering work on hormone-disrupting chemicals and persistent toxins. These authors have an excellent Website, which highlights ongoing battles to save our planet from the possible catastrophic effects of hormonal toxins. The Website is: www.ourstolenfuture.com

Lake Ontario Biomagnification of PCBs

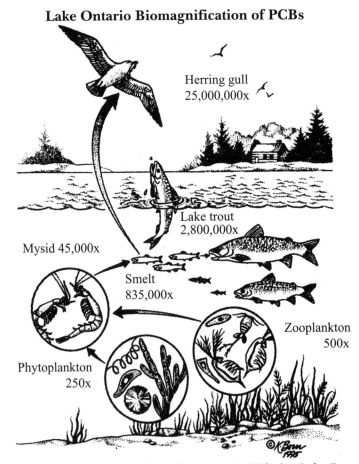

Source: Colborn, T., Dumanoski, D., and Myers, J. P. 1997. *Our Stolen Future: Are We Threatening Our Fertility, Intelligence, and Survival? A Scientific Detective Story.* New York, New York: Penguin. Reprinted with permission.

Swedish studies show that levels of PCBs in human breast milk have significantly declined in recent years. In countries that have not banned PCBs, levels remain high. Our main exposure comes from fat derived from animals near the top of the food chain. This fat is usually consumed in the form of fish, meat, or dairy products.[83] A half-life is defined as: "The time required for one-half of a quantity of a substance to be eliminated from a system." The half-life of the elimination of PCBs from animal fat is several decades.

Studies of Rhesus monkeys exposed to PCBs in the womb and through breast milk showed that they suffered impaired memory, learning, and motor skills. The higher their exposure, the more errors they made on cognitive tests. Hyperactivity has been reproduced in mice, rats, and monkeys exposed to PCBs in the womb and infancy. Men and women with occupational exposure to PCBs suffered an increased incidence of goiters and abnormalities of thyroid hormone levels.

In 1979, there was an accidental exposure to contaminated cooking oil in Taiwan. The oil had high levels of PCBs and furans. "Furans" are a family of toxins that are similar in structure and effect to dioxin (discussed later in this chapter). A medical study included 128 children who were either in the womb or conceived by women who were accidentally exposed to PCBs. Those born after the exposure were affected by residual contamination in the mother. Many of these children showed mild impairments in motor and mental abilities similar to those found in the animal studies. They also developed behavior problems including increased levels of activity and attention deficits. Their IQs averaged five points less than their unexposed peers. Exposed adult females had an increased incidence of goiters. However, their thyroid function blood tests did not differ markedly from the general population. In other human studies on PCB exposure, the thyroid function tests appear to be relatively unaffected as well. In contrast, many animal studies show numerous alterations in thyroid hormone tests, reflecting inhibition of thyroid function after exposure to PCBs.[80,81,82]

PCBs are a major contaminant in fish from the Great Lakes. Women contaminated with PCBs from eating these fish were studied over 15 years to see how it affected their children. Mothers who ate the most fish tended to have babies with lower birth weights and smaller head circumferences. Signs of neurological impairment in children with even slightly elevated levels of PCBs became apparent. Their verbal and memory scores were lower at four years of age. At age 11, the average IQ of children born to women with breast milk fat levels above 1.25 parts per million (ppm) was six points below those children from less contaminated mothers. In addition, these children were more distractible and had lower verbal comprehension scores. Women from the industrialized world average one part per million (ppm) in their breast milk fat. Developmental impairment from PCBs in other United States studies seems to correlate more with exposure in the womb than with lactation.[81,92]

Studies of rats exposed to PCBs in the womb added further evidence of impaired thyroid function. The fact that hypothyroidism may result in hearing loss and deafness was demonstrated in these rats, as they suffered hearing losses that were reversed by giving thyroid hormone.[81]

Dioxins

Dioxins (polychlorinated dibenzo-para-dioxins) and furans (polychlorinated dibenzofurans) are two closely related groups of chemical by-products. Incinerations of municipal or hazardous (hospitals) waste and sewage sludge that contain chlorine are primary sources. They are also formed during the production of chlorine containing chemicals such as pesticides, polyvinyl chloride (PVC) plastics, paper pulp bleaching, and from diesel-engine exhaust. Volcanoes and forest fires release small amounts. Dioxins contaminated the majority of herbicides used during the 1960s and 1970s. In 1974, almost seven million pounds of the most commonly contaminated herbicide, named 2,4,5-T, was used for urban and agricultural weed control in America. Nineteen million gallons of Agent Orange, which contains 2,4,5-T and dioxin, were spayed in

Vietnam. There are 75 variant forms of dioxins and 135 variants of furans. Seventeen of the most studied and toxic dioxins and furans are loosely referred to as "dioxin".

Like other persistent organic pollutants (POPs), dioxins are distributed throughout our planet's air, water, soil, sediment, food, and animals. Biomagnification results in concentration of the toxins at the top of the food chain. Our primary sources of exposure to dioxins are meat, dairy, and fish. Dioxins are stored in fat and easily penetrate the placenta. The half-life for their elimination from our fat is estimated to be seven years (half will be gone in seven years if no further accumulation occurs).

Dioxins are among the most hazardous of our ubiquitous chemical pollutants. They have been shown to be potent cancer-causing chemicals. Hodgkin's disease, non-Hodgkin's lymphoma, and soft tissue sarcomas are cancers linked to dioxin exposure in humans. Dioxins are thousands of times more toxic than arsenic to guinea pigs. Adult humans are more resistant to dioxins' poisonous effects. Dioxins have been shown to disrupt thyroid, testosterone, and estrogen functions in laboratory animals. Dosages of dioxin required to disrupt thyroid hormones in laboratory rats are 1,000 times less than those needed for PCBs. Animal studies suggest dioxins have the ability to inhibit thyroid function. Rats developed goiters after long-term low-dose exposure. A single dose of dioxin would lower the body temperature and basal metabolism in a young developing rat despite only having mild effects on its thyroid hormone blood level. This interference with thyroid metabolism is another illustration of Type 2 hypothyroidism. Abnormalities in the reproductive glands of both male and female offspring resulted when pregnant rats were given one extremely small dose of dioxin. Prenatal exposure to dioxin resulted in sharply reduced sperm counts in males rats and caused malformations in the female reproductive tracts.

Contrastingly, it has been shown that dioxins can over-stimulate thyroid function in other animal studies. Without thyroid hormones, tadpoles never develop into frogs. In one study, it was shown that tadpoles exposed to dioxin developed more rapidly than usual into frogs. In another study, mice pups and rat pups demonstrated enhanced spatial learning. The dioxin apparently facilitated the actions of thyroid hormones on the brain. The developing fetus is extremely sensitive to miniscule fluctuations in hormone levels, and far-reaching consequences can result.[81]

Research pioneered in the late 1970s by the American research scientist, Fred vom Saal, Ph.D., revealed precisely how sensitive prenatal mice were to fluctuations in estrogen or testosterone levels. The position of the fetal mouse in the womb caused minute fluctuations in hormone levels. If a female has been situated between two other females (exposing her to more estrogen and less testosterone), she ultimately would become more attractive to males, came into heat more often, and would be less aggressive than sisters who were situated between males inside their mother's womb. Females positioned between two males became much more aggressive and less likely to breed. They had been exposed to more testosterone and less estrogen. Dr. vom Saal proved the differences in traits resulted from tiny fluctuations in estrogen and testosterone in the developing fetus. These hormones had leached across from the neighboring fetus. A difference of 35 parts per trillion in exposure to estrogen and one part per billion in testosterone resulted in myriad life-long behavioral and physical changes in genetically identical mice. Many of the environmental toxins affect estrogen and testosterone in addition to thyroid functions.[82]

Times Beach, Missouri made national headlines in 1982, when oil, contaminated with dioxins, was sprayed on the city's dirt roads to control the dust. Floods spread the contamination throughout the town. All 2,240 residents were relocated. Children who were born later showed evidence of immune system abnormalities and brain dysfunction. Other studies showed dioxins lowered the sperm count and suppressed immune function in exposed men.

DDT

DDT and its derivatives are insecticides. DDT was introduced in 1939 and thought to be relatively safe. It was the most powerful insecticide ever discovered and the inventor was awarded the Nobel Prize. American soldiers in World War II were routinely de-loused with DDT. DDT became available for commercial use in 1945. By 1950, DDT was being spread across the land on farms, lawns, gardens, and suburban streets as an insecticide and part of mosquito control efforts. I have encountered many people who chased the trucks that sprayed DDT for mosquito control. When my mother saw the trucks, she closed all of our windows and doors and kept us inside.

Rachel Carson, a marine biologist for the U.S. Fish and Wildlife Service, published *Silent Spring* in 1962. The book chronicled the contamination of the entire world's food supply with DDT, the concentration of DDT and its derivatives in the fatty tissue of animals including humans, the resultant genetic damage, cancer, and the extinction of entire species.

After laboratory mice exposed to DDT developed cancers, further production was halted in America in 1972. Despite the ban, America produced over 96 tons of DDT for export overseas in 1991. DDT is still widely used to control mosquitoes that spread malaria in third world countries. Developing countries now harbor much higher levels of DDT than the United States. Average breast milk concentrations have decreased significantly in developed countries. The longer the time elapsed since being banned, the lower the concentrations found in breast milk.

DDT is broken down or metabolized into DDD and DDE. Unfortunately, DDD and DDE are just as persistent and toxic as DDT. Their half-life is about 57 years in a temperate environment and four to six years in our fat. DDT and its metabolites all interfere with the metabolism of thyroid hormones. Studies have shown that exposure causes goiters in rats. DDT also blocks testosterone receptors and interferes with estrogen hormones. Measurable levels of DDT, DDD, and DDE are still detectable in every man, woman, and child. These toxins cross the placenta and are transferred via breast milk.

HCB

Hexachlorobenzene (HCB) is a fungicide and an industrial by-product. It was widely used on grains and onions until its use as a fungicide was banned in the U.S. in 1965. It continues to be produced as an industrial by-product in chlorination processes such as wastewater treatment and in the manufacture of solvents like carbon tetrachloride. HCB and its metabolites are also widely distributed and biomagnified. Food from contaminated soils, fish from contaminated waters, and milk or meat from animals that graze on contaminated land are major sources of HCB. Our drinking water harbors small amounts. HCBs are stored in fat and easily cross the placenta.

The main breakdown product, or metabolite, of HCB has marked thyroid effects. In 1955, between 3,000 and 4,000 Turkish people were accidentally poisoned with grain contaminated with HCB. Two to three decades later, 59% of women and 23% of men had developed goiters among a group of 225 survivors. HCB has been shown to cause goiters, thyroid tumors, and decreased thyroid hormone production in hamsters. Rats developed hormone profiles consistent with hypothyroidism after exposure to HCB.

Aminotriazole

Aminotriazole (amitrole) is an extensively used herbicide. It is employed in weed control before planting and after harvesting. Amitrole is not a persistent organic pollutant in the soil. However, its residues are absorbed by commercially grown food. In 2003, Northern Ireland enacted laws governing maximum allowable residue levels of amitrole and other common herbicides and pesticides in their foodstuffs.

Studies of amitrole have clearly shown that it causes Type 1 hypothyroidism and goiters in rats and other rodents. Its propensity to cause goiters is so strong that it is used in many experimental studies on rodents to investigate goiters.

As discussed in Chapter 5, goiters were recognized as one of the first symptoms of hypothyroidism in the early nineteenth century. Chemicals that cause goiters are termed "goitrogens". In her research article on synthetic thyroid toxins, Dr. Brucker-Davis correctly stated, "The respective role of natural and synthetic goitrogens is often difficult to sort out. The impact on humans may depend on timing, dose, and duration of exposure, synergy between chemicals, as well as genetic and immune status predisposing the exposed person to thyroid disease." The same principles hold true for synthetic and natural toxins and their ability to produce Type 2 hypothyroidism.[35]

Phthalates

Phthalates (pronounced thal-eights) are a large group of synthetic industrial chemicals. Worldwide annual production is estimated to be about one billion pounds per year. Their most common use is to soften plastics and make them flexible. As much as half of the mass of a soft plastic container can be phthalates. Industrial usages include hair spray additives, dyes, cosmetics, adhesives, oily perfumes, and lubricants. In 1998, manufacturers of baby pacifiers, toys, and medical supplies were asked to remove the most toxic phthalates from their products by the U.S. Consumer Product Safety Commission.

These chemicals readily leach into fluids contained by the plastic. Drinking water and soda are easily contaminated. Edible oils stored in plastic and microwave oven food cooked or warmed in plastic containers are particularly contaminated. **Phthalates interfere with thyroid hormone metabolism and adversely affect testosterone function**. The good news is that they are cleared from the body within a few days of exposure. The bad news is that, as you can imagine, an incredible number of people are being exposed on a daily basis. Studies from the U.S. Centers for Disease Control show this widespread human exposure.

Male rats suffered reproductive-system birth defects when exposed to phthalates during the first trimester. An Italian study found a common phthalate in 88% of the samples from umbilical cord blood taken from 84 consecutive newborns. Babies found to have phthalates were 50% more likely to be born prematurely and averaged 38 weeks gestation versus 39 weeks for the babies without phthalates. Recall that premature births are associated with Type 2 hypothyroidism. Another study from scientists at the CDC and Harvard showed adult men with high levels of phthalates were much more likely to have low sperm motility and decreased sperm counts. In 2003, the American Academy of Pediatrics recommended research on phthalates' effects on the fetus and infants.[84,85]

Phthalates are used in many synthetic surgical implants. In America, breast implants for enhancement increased from 32,000 in 1992 to over 225,000 in 2002. Another 70,000 breast implants for surgical reconstruction were also performed in 2002. Increased fatigue, muscle aches, and hair loss were found in many patients several years after their implants. Fatigue, muscle aches, and hair loss are among the most common symptoms of hypothyroidism. Increased age was given as a possible explanation for these symptoms. A more likely explanation is phthalate-induced exacerbation of Type 2 hypothyroidism. As previously noted, thyroid hormones are chiefly responsible for development of the sex glands. Underdeveloped breasts are a common manifestation of Type 2 hypothyroidism.

The following pictures illustrate the potential for improving a female's breasts and genitalia. Drs. Lisser and Escamilla termed this type of hypothyroidism, "adolescent hypothyroidism with infantilism".[48] See page 214 for descriptions of the pictures on the next page.

Fig. 1a   Fig. 1b

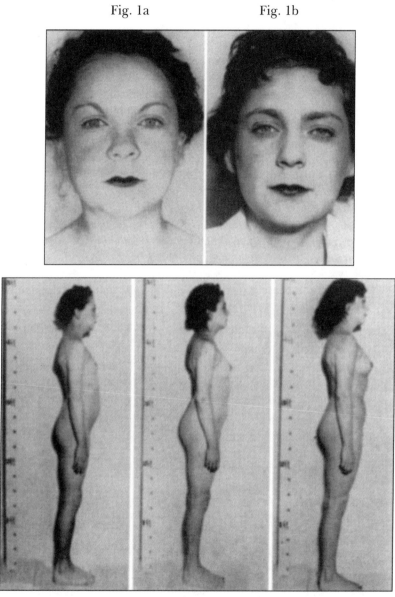

Fig. 1c   Fig. 1d   Fig. 1e

Source: Lisser, H., and Escamilla, R. F. *Atlas of Clinical Endocrinology: Including Text of Diagnosis and Treatment.* C.V. Mosby Company, 1957. Reprinted with permission.

Figure 1a shows the appearance of the 27 year-old woman's face before treatment with desiccated thyroid. She had puffiness around her nose and eyes but had no overt myxedema (according to the authors). Her menses began at age 16 and were irregular with scant flow. She had no interest in the opposite sex. There was an absence of pubic hair. She was constipated, gained weight easily, had dry skin and hair, had anemia, and she tired easily. Her heart rate was 58, blood pressure was 98/70, BMR was minus 27%, and her bone age was 14 on X-rays.

Figure 1b shows the patient's face after 10 months of taking desiccated thyroid. She was about to be married. BMR was minus 5%. Her anemia was resolving. Her periods were every 25 or 26 days and her flow had improved.

Figure 1c shows the side body profile of the same patient before treatment. The breasts had not developed and there was no hair on the arms or legs. Her height was 4 feet 11 inches.

Figure 1d shows the patient after 10 months of thyroid therapy. Her breasts had enlarged.

Figure 1e shows the same patient 13 months later. She was taking 2 grains of desiccated thyroid. One mg of stilbesterol (synthetic estrogen) had been added. Her breasts and pelvis had enlarged further. Her libido and gratification increased.

Common Heavy Metal Toxins: Lead, Arsenic, and Mercury

Mitochondria contain enzymes that are crucial for the production of our bodies' energy molecules. A group of these crucial enzymes are particularly sensitive to the effects of heavy metals. In addition to impeding the function of mitochondria, heavy metals directly poison or interfere with other critical enzymes and thyroid functions.

The following two examples illustrate the pervasive nature of these metals in our environment. A study was done on a 13 year-old girl with a history of recurrent staph infections. Her medical history was typical of Type 2 hypothyroidism. The patient had no known exposures to any hazardous materials. Yet, at 13, she already had accumulated noticeable levels of arsenic, lead, cadmium, nickel, antimony, titanium, as well as elevated levels of aluminum. She enjoyed surfing in the ocean. Our oceans are now contaminated with heavy metals and numerous toxins. Whether or not these toxic metals contributed to her chronic infections is up for debate. Regardless, we know that heavy metals disrupt thyroid metabolism as well as many of the enzyme reactions throughout the body. Her elevated level of copper was probably due to her shampoo or a form of copper used as a fungicide in swimming pools. A sample of her hair was used for the test. This patient also had mercury contamination. A minority of people are unable to eliminate any mercury through their hair and called "nonexcretors".

> Small amounts of several heavy metals including chromium, zinc, copper, manganese, and selenium also play essential roles for normal physiological functions.

Potentially Toxic Elements

TOXIC ELEMENTS	RESULT µg/g	REFERENCE RANGE	PERCENTILE 68th	95th
Arsenic	0.04	< 0.14		
Lead	0.5	< 4.0		
Mercury	< 0.03	< 3.0		
Cadmium	0.074	< 0.5		
Chromium	0.36	< 0.7		
Beryllium	< 0.01	< 0.05		
Cobalt	0.062	< 0.15		
Nickel	0.7	< 1.0		
Zinc	160	< 300		
Copper	160	< 65		
Thorium	0.001	< 0.01		
Thallium	< 0.001	< 0.02		
Barium	0.25	< 8.0		
Cesium	< 0.002	< 0.01		
Manganese	0.29	< 1.5		
Selenium	0.72	< 2.7		
Bismuth	0.1	< 0.35		
Vanadium	0.1	< 0.2		
Silver	0.25	< 0.9		
Antimony	0.04	< 0.12		
Palladium	< 0.004	< 0.01		
Aluminum	27	< 19		
Platinum	< 0.003	< 0.01		
Tungsten	< 0.01	< 0.02		
Tin	0.43	< 0.8		
Uranium	0.02	< 0.2		
Gold	0.03	< 0.4		
Tellurium	< 0.05	< 0.05		
Germanium	0.05	< 0.085		
Titanium	1.1	< 2.0		
Gadolinium	0.005	< 0.008		
Total Toxic Exposure Index				

µg/g = parts per million

The next study is that of a 53 year-old former steel mill worker who is an electrician. His test reflects how heavy metals may accumulate to dangerous levels from daily exposures.

Potentially Toxic Elements

TOXIC ELEMENTS	RESULT µg/g	REFERENCE RANGE	PERCENTILE 68th	95th
Arsenic	0.16	< 0.4		
Lead	2.5	< 8.0		
Mercury	0.99	< 3.0		
Cadmium	3.3	< 0.7		
Chromium	2.2	< 0.75		
Beryllium	< 0.01	< 0.05		
Cobalt	0.16	< 0.15		
Nickel	2.9	< 1.0		
Zinc	210	< 350		
Copper	19	< 50		
Thorium	< 0.001	< 0.01		
Thallium	0.002	< 0.02		
Barium	8.8	< 6.0		
Cesium	0.004	< 0.01		
Manganese	2.6	< 1.5		
Selenium	1.6	< 2.7		
Bismuth	0.074	< 0.22		
Vanadium	0.098	< 0.3		
Silver	0.06	< 0.6		
Antimony	0.21	< 0.25		
Palladium	< 0.004	< 0.01		
Aluminum	36	< 30		
Platinum	< 0.003	< 0.01		
Tungsten	0.017	< 0.02		
Tin	0.31	< 0.8		
Uranium	0.002	< 0.2		
Gold	0.01	< 0.4		
Tellurium	< 0.05	< 0.05		
Germanium	0.065	< 0.085		
Titanium	2.7	< 2.0		
Gadolinium	< 0.001	< 0.008		
Total Toxic Exposure Index				

SPECIMEN DATA

µg/g = parts per million

He suffered from Type 2 hypothyroidism, chronic pain, fatigue, and recurrent upper respiratory infections. Eighteen months of expensive and time-consuming treatments greatly reduced his burden of toxic metals. The combination of thyroid hormones and detoxification alleviated most of his other symptoms as well.

Lead

Recently, the Centers for Disease Control (CDC) estimated approximately 400,000 American children, over 2% of our children, had dangerous levels of lead in their blood. Twenty years earlier, the CDC had estimated that over 80% of our children were affected. In spite of the marked improvement, exposure to lead remains one of the most serious environmental threats facing expectant mothers and children.

Most of Europe had banned white leaded paint by 1930. Despite overwhelming evidence of the dangers posed by lead, the American lead industry successfully forestalled a ban on leaded paint until 1978. Soil concentrations are especially high around older homes due to paint remnants and dust. Leaded gasoline wasn't banned until 1985. Motor vehicles' exhaust aerosolized the lead, which tended to settle in the soil around busy streets. Front yards remain more contaminated than back yards.

The Agency for Toxic Substances and Disease Registry (ATSDR) of the U.S. Department of Health and Human Services estimated that three million tons of lead derived from paint and four million tons of lead derived from leaded gasoline remain in paint on old homes, paint dust, and our soil. Lead is still legally used in American batteries, vinyl, stained glass, bullets, and many imported products. Neighborhoods downwind from lead smelters are thoroughly contaminated. Lead soldered copper pipes or solid lead pipes in the plumbing of old homes are common sources of lead poisoning. Dangerous levels of lead may be found in calcium supplements made from bone meal and oyster shells. China, ceramic cookware, and crystal may leach lead into food or drink. Cigarette smoke contains lead. Renovation of old homes frequently exposes the occupants to lead. Old water cooler fountains in schools often were lined with lead. They were recalled in 1988, yet many continue to poison our children. *Lead Is a Silent Hazard* is an excellent book about the detection, treatment, and prevention of lead poisoning.[86]

Lead is stored in our bones and teeth. The half-life for elimination in humans is 13 years. The stored lead is mobilized during pregnancy and easily crosses the placenta. Lead profoundly interferes with the developing brain. Low-level lead poisoning can result in reading and learning disabilities, reduced memory and intelligence, irritability, attention deficit disorders, and hyperactivity. Other complications include anemia, kidney damage, delayed developmental milestones, problems with balance, and a multitude of social and behavioral problems. Interference with thyroid functions has been documented in children.[81,87]

Dr. Herbert Needleman studied 12,000 children in Boston, Massachusetts, comparing the amount of lead found in their baby teeth with their performance in school. The students' success was inversely related to their lead levels. Children with higher lead levels (20 parts per billion) were six times more likely to have reading disabilities, vocabulary deficits, problems with attention, loss of fine motor coordination, and an average IQ of four to six points below their less toxic peers. **A four point lowering of IQ scores translates into a 50% increase in the number of retarded children.** Lead toxicity has been associated with increased disciplinary problems, including violent behavior in juvenile and adult males.[86]

The CDC now considers blood levels of 10 parts per billion (ppb) to be dangerous. The average lead levels in children have declined from 15 ppb to 4 ppb in the last 20 years. Current CDC estimates of lead toxicity are at 22% for urban African-American children and 13% for urban Mexican-American children.

A 2003 research study published in *The New England Journal of Medic*ine showed that no amount of lead is safe. They concluded that blood lead levels were inversely related to children's IQ scores. **IQ declined by over seven points as lifetime average blood lead concentrations increased from 1 to 10 ppb**. These low levels were previously thought to be "safe". The researchers concluded that many more U.S. children might be adversely affected by environmental lead than had been previously estimated.[88]

Proposals to clean urban housing of leaded paint and contamination were put forth in the United States Congress and Senate. Public apathy and lack of funding are reasons given for our failure to begin such programs.

Arsenic

Arsenic is ubiquitous in our food, water, soil, and air. It is a by-product of the smelting process for metal ores such as copper, lead, gold, zinc, cobalt, and nickel. Combustion of fossil fuels, the manufacturing of glass and electronic components such as semiconductors, diodes, and photoelectric cells all contribute. Wood preservatives, paints, and pigments often contain arsenic.

Most human exposure comes from pesticides, herbicides, and fungicides that end up in our food and water. The Agency for Toxic Substances and Disease Registry (ATSDR) estimates the average American's dietary intake of arsenic is between 11 and 14 micrograms per day. Meat, fish, and poultry are responsible for the majority of this intake. Grapes and tobacco are frequently sprayed with arsenic-containing pesticides, which exposes humans to arsenic from wine and tobacco products.

Arsenic accumulates in the hair, nails, skin, bone, the gastrointestinal tract, and the thyroid gland. Arsenic is a major antagonist of selenium, an essential mineral in our diet. Critical enzymes responsible for thyroid hormone metabolism are dependent upon selenium. Arsenic is known to cause goiters and readily crosses the placenta. Increased frequency of spontaneous abortions and birth defects have been linked to arsenic. It also interferes with many other critical biochemical and enzyme reactions that are necessary to maintain health. Therefore, many different organs are adversely affected.

Arsenic is strongly associated with lung and skin cancers and has been linked to several other forms of cancer. Chronic toxicity may result in weakness, aching muscles, gastrointestinal upset, and peripheral neuropathies (nerve damage resulting in loss of sensation and atrophy or weakness of muscles in the feet and lower legs).

Under the United States Freedom of Information Act, The National Resources Defense Council (NRDC) obtained data compiled by the Environmental Protection Agency (EPA) on the amount of contamination from arsenic in our drinking water. Over 100,000 samples from more than 24,000 public water systems in 25 states, collected between 1980 and 1998, were analyzed for arsenic. The following chart represents the data collected from the states where samples were taken.

National Arsenic Occurrence Map

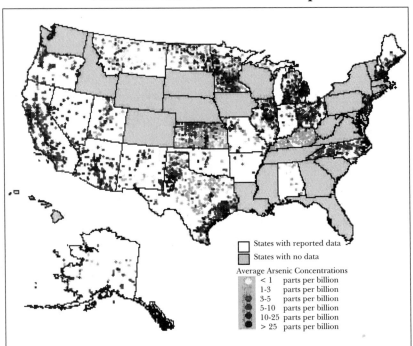

Source: National Resources Defense Council (NRDC.org). 2003. National Arsenic Occurrence Map. Retrieved from Internet October 31, 2003 at: http://www.nrdc.org/water/drinking/arsenic/map.asp

After a decade of public hearings and scientific reviews, the EPA set a limit of 10 parts per billion (ppb) as the allowable level of arsenic in public drinking water. The EPA and the National Academy of Sciences concluded that chronic exposure to arsenic resulted in an increased risk of cancer. The current standard of 50 ppb was set in 1942.

Several years ago, the World Health Organization and the European Union implemented the 10 ppb standard. The U.S. limit of 10 ppb was to be implemented on January 1, 2001. Unfortunately, the new standard has yet to be implemented. The estimated cost to reduce arsenic in drinking water to desirable levels is less than three dollars per month for families living in areas with high levels of arsenic.

Mercury

Mercury ranks highly among the most poisonous threats to animal life. It is also ubiquitous in our air, food, and water. Annual worldwide emissions of mercury are estimated to be 2,200 metric tons. One-third of the emissions are from natural sources such as volcanoes and the decay of sediments containing mercury. Combustion of fossil fuels accounts for 25% of the total. In developed countries, medical waste incineration contributes a large percentage. In the U.S., coal-fired power plants are responsible for one-third of the total atmospheric emissions. The following chart represents the latest figures on atmospheric emissions from the EPA.

Up In Smoke: Breakdown of mercury emissions in the U.S., 1994-95*

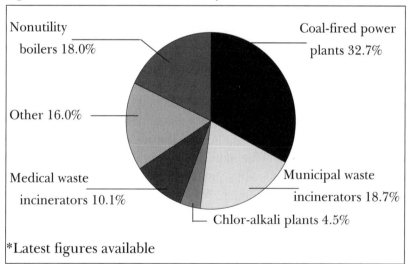

Nonutility boilers 18.0%

Coal-fired power plants 32.7%

Other 16.0%

Medical waste incinerators 10.1%

Municipal waste incinerators 18.7%

Chlor-alkali plants 4.5%

*Latest figures available

Source: U.S. EPA Mercury Study Report to Congress.

Mercury, in the form of thimerosal, has been used as a preservative in vaccinations for decades. In 2003, my doctor offered a tetanus booster as part of a routine physical exam. I was appalled to learn it contained thimerosal. Having undergone several years of aggressive treatment to eliminate the reservoir of mercury that had accumulated in my body, I declined the shot. I had mistakenly believed thimerosal was finally phased out.

The use of mercury has declined in fungicides and pesticides, but soil residues persist and find their way into the food chain. Auto exhaust, drinking water, processed foods, mascara, mercurochrome and merthiolate, floor waxes and polishes, adhesives, latex paint made prior to 1991, and wood preservatives are other possible sources of exposure.

Among all of the pollutants listed in the EPA Mercury Study, mercury was the only one for which levels are not dropping. The report warned that emissions of mercury from coal-fired power plants and from other industrial sources pose a serious health risk. The EPA study estimated that at least 8% of American women of childbearing age have blood levels of mercury that represent a "higher risk of adverse health effects" to a fetus. Their estimate may be low. Blood levels and hair samples were taken from women and children in their study. These samples may not reveal the true burden of mercury contamination. Mercury promptly binds with body tissues, and our level of mercury may be higher than the levels indicated by hair and blood tests. Once mercury is bound to other tissues, it may leach very slowly into the bloodstream. Hair analysis may provide a slightly more accurate estimate for levels of lead, arsenic, and mercury due to chronic exposure. It, too, may be misleadingly low for heavy metal tests. Injecting certain chemicals that bind or "chelate" heavy metals is a more accurate test. The urine is collected following the injection and the excreted metals are measured. There are no easy methods for accurately estimating mercury burden levels.

Mercury easily crosses the placenta. The most deleterious effects are to fetuses and infants. One of the scientists who authored the EPA study stated, "Putting as much mercury in the biosphere as we do is something we're going to regret, I think, for a long, long time."[89]

Mercury is biomagnified, and high levels are often found in fish. As of 2002, there were 1,782 advisories (one per body of water) issued by the EPA in 41 states restricting the consumption of fish or shellfish due to their mercury content. Sixteen states had issued statewide or statewide coastal advisories.

The World Health Organization states that the highest mercury exposure to humans currently comes from dental

amalgam fillings. More than 100 million of these fillings are placed each year in the U.S. **The silver amalgams used for dental cavities are 50% mercury**, 35% silver, and 15% of the total is a mixture of tin, copper, and zinc. These amalgams constantly emit mercury vapors that are absorbed. Various laboratories have estimated the average daily body absorption from amalgam ranges between 1.2 and 27 micrograms per day. **The World Health Organization estimates the average to be at 23 micrograms per day for individuals with five or more fillings**. Research has shown that the amount of mercury in subjects' blood and feces directly correlates with their total amalgam surface area. Human autopsy studies reveal significantly higher mercury concentrations in the brain and kidneys of subjects with aged amalgams than in subjects with no mercury fillings.[64]

Mercury is particularly toxic to the nervous system, especially the developing brain. Potential effects on the fetal brain include inhibition of thyroid metabolism as well as direct damage to the developing nerve cells.

Damage to the mitochondria, inhibition of mitochondrial enzymes, suppression of protein synthesis, and the production of free radicals are physiological consequences of mercury and arsenic toxicity. The combination of lead and mercury has a synergistic effect, multiplying their potential for damage.[90] The former Chairman of The University of Kentucky's Department of Chemistry, Dr. Boyd Haley, established a link between Alzheimer's disease and exposure to mercury.[96]

Early signs of mercury toxicity include decreased senses of vision, hearing, touch, and taste; a metallic taste in the mouth, fatigue or lack of physical endurance, and increased salivation. Symptoms may progress to include anorexia (i.e., decreased appetite), numbness, paresthesias (abnormal sensations such as burning or prickling of the skin), headaches, high blood pressure, irritability, excitability, and immune suppression. Consequences from more advanced poisoning may include: tremors, incoordination, anemia, psychosis, manic behavior, autoimmune disorders, and kidney failure. Proper treatment of hypothyroidism may offer significant protection against these deleterious effects.

Lead, arsenic, and mercury are the three most frequently found toxic substances in America according to the Agency for Toxic Substances and Disease Registry (ATSDR) of the U.S. Department of Health and Human Services. These figures come from the U.S. government's Priority List of Hazardous Substances.

I never witnessed one test for chronic heavy metal toxicity in a patient during all of my formal medical training. The diagnostic paradigms did not include heavy metal toxicity.

> The International College of Integrative Medicine (www.icimed.com) and The American College for Advancement in Medicine (www.acam.org) offer listings of doctors who offer treatment for metal toxicity.

Brief Overview of Environmental Illnesses:
Symptoms and Treatment

Thirty years of extensive research on tens of thousands of environmentally ill patients has been performed at the Environmental Health Center of Dallas (EHCD). William Rea M.D., is the founder and director of this world-renowned clinic. He is a cardiovascular surgeon and serves on the Board of Directors of the American Academy of Environmental Medicine and also the American Environmental Health Foundation. The remarkable successes of Dr. Rea's clinic shed light on the profound effect environmental toxins have on our population.

Thirty years ago, Dr. Rea developed severe chemical sensitivities while serving as chief of thoracic surgery at the Veterans Hospital and Clinical Associate Professor of Thoracic Surgery at The University of Texas Southwestern Medical School. He sought help from medical pioneers in the budding new field of environmental medicine. The magnitude and breadth of medical problems associated with environmental medicine captivated him and became his life's work.

Chemical sensitivity is an adverse reaction to ambient levels of toxic chemicals contained in air, food, and water. The nature of the reaction depends upon an individual's susceptibility, the chemical nature of the substance, the tissues or organs involved in the reaction, and several other factors such as duration of exposure and the patient's nutritional status. For example, many people suffer headaches when exposed to ambient levels of perfume or cigarette smoke.

Dr. Rea's clinic provides a uniquely controlled environment. The air, water, and food are free of synthetic chemicals. Many patients' symptoms markedly improve soon after being placed in the pollution-free environment. Patients undergo a battery of tests including fat biopsies to determine their toxic burden. Nutritional status is evaluated. Tests are performed to determine environmentally related illnesses such as chemical sensitivities and allergies to molds or foods. Treatment for these problems begins after the initial testing.

Research by Dr. Rea and his staff at the EHCD has shown that pollutant overload is particularly deleterious to three of our most critical physiological systems. The immune system, nervous system, and endocrine system are frequent targets of pollutants. The end result is an epidemic of chronic illnesses. The same three systems are also favorite targets of hypothyroidism.

Many maladies are common to both pollutant injury and hypothyroidism. In fact, there is a recurring theme of underlying hypothyroidism present in the population of chemically sensitive patients treated at Dr. Rea's clinic as well as mine. Genetic predisposition, low body temperature, muscle weakness, low energy, poor circulation, inability to perspire, constipation, multiple endocrine problems, as well as numerous other symptoms are common to pollutant injury and hypothyroidism. A majority of these patients are women and children. Women and children are more severely affected by hypothyroidism. Dr. Rea's research has shown that pollutants often stimulate the tissues responsible for immunity. Many chemically sensitive patients exhibit increased immune function. Another group suffers impaired immunity and recurrent viral, bacterial, or fungal infections. Many of these symptoms resolve after treatment for environmentally related illnesses or with thyroid hormones or both. The logical conclusion is that pollutants often target thyroid metabolism. Those affected with Type 2 hypothyroidism appear to be more susceptible to the deleterious effects of pollutants.

Neurotransmitters send chemical messages from nerves to the target cells or to other nerves. Scientific research has elucidated the tremendous influence thyroid hormones have on neurotransmitters. These interactions are complex and not fully understood. However, research indicates thyroid hormones regulate a plethora of different neurotransmitters by potentiating the effects of each of these chemical messengers. Neurotransmitters both stimulate and inhibit physiological activity. The ability of thyroid hormones to both stimulate and inhibit chemical messengers provides an explanation for the dichotomous effects of hypothyroidism and environmental thyroid toxins. As previously mentioned, dioxins appear to both stimulate and suppress thyroid hormone actions in different animal studies. The same holds true regarding hypothyroidism and its affects on humankind. For instance, puberty may be premature or delayed. The sex glands may become over-developed or under-developed. Growth may be stunted or exaggerated. People may be sluggish or hyperactive.[91]

I believe our genetic tendency toward Type 2 hypothyroidism is now epidemic. This predisposition, combined with prenatal and postnatal exposure to pervasive hormone toxins, is largely responsible for the explosion of chronic physical and mental illnesses in Western Civilization. Thirty-five years ago, Dr. Barnes predicted the epidemic of heart disease, diabetes, and other chronic illnesses linked with hypothyroidism. I have outlined the research he used to prove his point. Today, his predictions have been realized. Many chemical sensitivities are also linked to hypothyroidism, and their incidence will likely mushroom.

Under Attack: Environmental Medical Treatment

Dr. Rea and many other physicians are being attacked by their state medical boards who are acting under pressure from insurance companies to disallow the practice of environmental medicine. This is an exhaustive and costly endeavor for Dr. Rea who continues to champion our right for access to appropriate and effective treatment for chemical sensitivity and injury. A legal defense fund has been created to fight this injustice. To see the complete letter from Dr. Rea's office and where to contribute see Appendix C.

Table 12.1 Commercial Food[a] vs Less Chemically Contaminated Food[b]

Food	Organic: Less chemically contaminated foods (private survey)[a]		Chemically contaminated commercial foods (private survey) one market[b]		Commercial foods (EPA survey) multiple markets[c]	
	Pesticide	ppm	Pesticide	ppm	Pesticide	ppm
Beef	None	0	Trimethyl/parathion	Tr	Multiple	+
Pork	Endrin	Tr	Dicldrin/endrin	0.80	Multiple	+
Broccoli	Aidrin	Tr	Lindane	0.15	Dacthal	0.01
Cabbage	None	0	Lindane	1.13	Lindane	+
Carrot	None	0	None	0.33	Botran	1.10
				0	Trifluralin	0.01-0.15
					DDE	0.03-0.12
					Endrin	0.01
					Dieldrin	0.01
					DDT	0.03
Watercress	None	0	Not studied	—	Thiodin	2.55
Cauliflower	None	0	None	0	Lindane	0.01
Celery	None	0	None	0	Pesticide	+
Corn	None	0	None	0	Herbicide	+
					Fumigant	+
					Fensulfothion	+
					Imidan	+
Cucumber	None	0	None	0	Dieldrin	+
					DDE	0.01-0.03
					Endosulfan	0.04
					Diazinon	0.02
					Thiodan	4.10
					Aldicarb	0.05
					CIPC	0.01-0.17

Tr: trace amounts.

Table 12.1 cont. **Commercial Food[a] vs Less Chemically Contaminated Food[b]**

Food	Organic: Less chemically contaminated foods (private survey)[a]		Chemically contaminated commercial foods (private survey) one market[b]		Commercial foods (EPA survey) multiple markets[c]	
	Pesticide	ppm	Pesticide	ppm	Pesticide	ppm
Lettuce	None	0	None	0	DDE	0.01-0.03
					Endosulfan	0.04
					Diazinon	0.02
					Thiodan	4.10
					Aldicarb	0.05
Potato	None	0	None	0	CIPC	0.01-0.17
					Aldicarb	0.05
Spinach	None	0	Diazinon	0.48	CIPC	0.01-0.17
					DDT	0.02
					DDE	0.02-0.04
					Dacthal	0.02
Strawberry	None	0			Malanthion	0.01-0.21
					Endosulfan	0.14
					DDE	0.01-0.08
					Kelthane	0.07-3.70
					Mevinphos	0.02-0.28
String bean	None	0	Not done	monitor 0.91		
Apple	None	0	Not done	multiple +		
Avocado	None	0	Not done			
Banana	None	0	Not done			
Pear	None	0	Not done			
Tomato	None	0	Not done			
					Ethylene	+
					Pesticide	+
					Botran	0.77
					Fenvalerate	0.02
Beet (tops)	None	0			Dacthal	0.14

Table 12.1 cont.

Commercial Food^a vs Less Chemically Contaminated Food^b

Food	Organic: Less chemically contaminated foods (private survey)[a]		Chemically ceutamluated commercial foods (private survey) one market[b]		Commercial foods (EPA survey) multiple markets[c]	
	Pesticide	ppm	Pesticide	ppm	Pesticide	ppm
Orange	None	0			DDE	0.01
					Parathion	0.04
					Chlorpyrifos	0.01—0.12
					Ethion	0.19
					Kelthane	0.17—0.43
					Methidathion	0.05—0.53
					Fumigant	+
					Fenthion	0.5
					Fungicide	+
Oatmeal	None	0			Dacthal	1.43
					Monitor	1.78
					Diazinon	0.96
Rice	None	0			Daconil	123.00
Radish	None	0			Thiodan	0.69
Bell pepper	None	0	Not done		Bravo/Daconol	0.16
Collard green	None	0	Not done		Diazinon	2.16
Daikon	None	0	Not done		Dieldrin	0.01
Mushroom	None	0	Not done		Pesticide	+
Parsley	None	0	Not done		Pesticide	+
Eggplant	None	0	Not done			
Grape	None	0	Not done			

a Acquired through the EHC-Dallas less chemically contaminated network.
b Acquired at commercial grocery store.
c + = positive, but the number is unknown.

Source: Rea, W. 1992. *Chemical Sensitivity, Vol. 2, Sources of Total Body Load.* Lewis Publishers. Reprinted with permission.

Table 12.2   **Sources of Synthetic Contamination of
Food during Transportation, Storage, and Preparation**

Transportation:
    Containers   Oiled burlap sacks, plastic sacks, solid
                                          containers, fungicided cardboard boxes
    Insecticides   Spraying en route to prevent infestation
    Fuel exhausts   Animals breathing during transportation

Storage:
    Heat   Pasteurization — milk — loss of nutrients
    Gases for ripening   Ethylene — bananas, other fruits
    Waxing   Cucumbers, turnips, green peppers
    Fungicides   Grains, peanuts, strawberries
    Bleaching   Chlorine, sulfuric acid — French fried
                                          potatoes, asparagus, cut apples
    Containers   Phenols, plastics, pesticides — cans, boxes,
                                          bottles
    Sweeteners   Saccharin (sulfur), aspartane, refined sugar
    Colorings   Tartrazines, other dyes — yellow, blue, green
    Preservatives   Antibiotics, BHA,BHT, propyl gallate, sulfurs,
                                          salt, formaldehyde, nitrates, nitrites
                                    — dried fruit, bacon, packed goods, candies,
                                        other sweets, carrageenin
    Emulsifiers   Polysorbates
    Thickeners & stabilizers Guar gums, other gums
    Flavorings   Aldehydes — fruit flavors
    Extractors   Methylene chloride — decaffinateds; hexanes
                                        — vegetable oils
    Irradiation   Fruit juice, milk, potatoes, onions, pork

Preparation:
    Smoking and barbecuing with synthetic fuel or natural woods —
            benzapyrenes, nitrosoamines
    Gas, oil roasting and broiling — hydrocarbons
    Cookware — aluminum, plastic, copper
    Flavor enhancers — monosodium and monoammonium glutamate
    Baking powder — aluminum

Source: Rea, W. 1992. *Chemical Sensitivity, Vol. 2, Sources of Total Body Load.*
Lewis Publishers. Reprinted with permission.

Table 12.3

Comparison of Contaminants Identified in Drinking Water and Contaminants Found in the Blood of the Chemically Sensitive

	Drinking and bathing water analysis	Blood of chemically sensitive
Chlorinated pesticides:		
Aldrin	+	+
Dieldrin	+	+
Chlordane	+	+
Heptachlor epoxide	+	+
Trans nonachlor	+	+
Hexachloro benzene	+	+
Benzene hexachloride	+	+
Organophosphate pesticide	+	+
Organic solvents:	+	+
Chloroform	+	+
Tetrachloroethylene	+	+
Trichloroethylene	+	+
Trichloroethane	+	+
Dichloromethane	+	+
Benzene	+	+
Xylene	+	+
Toluene	+	+
Dimethyl benzene	+	+
Trimethyl benzene	+	+
Aluminum	+	+
Barium	+	+
Lead	+	+
Mercury	+	+

Source: Rea, W. 1992. *Chemical Sensitivity, Vol. 2, Sources of Total Body Load*. Lewis Publishers. Reprinted with permission.

Table 12.4   **Coriolis Effect**

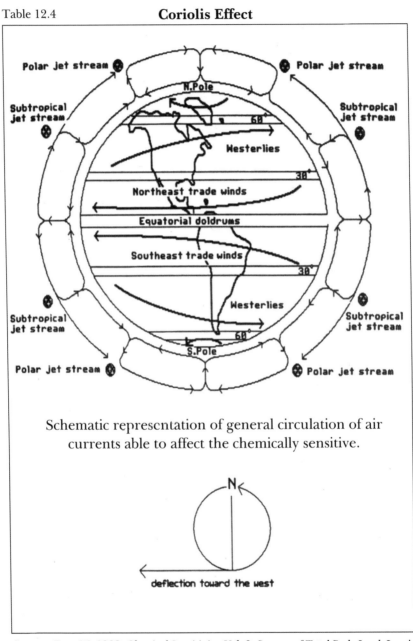

Schematic representation of general circulation of air
currents able to affect the chemically sensitive.

Source: Rea, W. 1992. *Chemical Sensitivity, Vol. 2, Sources of Total Body Load*. Lewis
Publishers. Reprinted with permission.

Table 12.5

Sources of Pollutants in Outside Air

Toxic air chemical release by industry (EPA)

Industry	Pounds/year	Industry	Pounds/year	Industry	Pounds/year
Chemicals	886,571,603	Printing & publishing	47,002,058	Food	15,651,659
Primary Metal	215,100,461	Machinery, exc. Elect.	46,242,666	Leather	13,783,466
Paper	207,880,906	Furniture and fixtures	45,252,222	Tobacco	7,460,460
Transportation Equip.	192,046,240	Instruments	41,622,386	Apparel	2,092,960
Rubber and plastics	132,037,605	Textiles	34,916,077	Multiple categories	184,786,760
Fabricated metals	110,227,308	Stone, clay, and glass	25,690,460	Non-manufacturing	32,751,890
Elec./electronic equip.	89,709,015	Lumber and wood	24,986,722		
Petroleum & coal prod.	75,513,067	Misc. manufacturing	21,748,310	Total	2,453,074,931

Air toxic chemicals by state (in rank order)

State	Emissions	State	Emissions	State	Emissions
Texas	229,910,640	Kentucky	43,279,655	Rhode Island	17,170,133
Louisiana	134,524,442	Missouri	43,151,138	Arizona	15,031,406
Tennessee	132,461,157	Arkansas	42,832,699	Nebraska	13,698,725
Virginia	131,359,106	Washington	39,893,330	New Hampshire	13,086,835
Ohio	122,464,629	New Jersey	38,631,572	Maine	11,624,580
Michigan	106,236,445	Iowa	36,208,159	Colorado	8,911,711
Indiana	103,479,027	Florida	35,354,199	Montana	5,032,798
Illinois	103,093,458	Alaska	31,707,083	Idaho	4,066,590
Georgia	94,296,297	West Virginia	31,582,771	Delaware	3,181,998
North Carolina	92,328,287	Minnesota	29,031,436	Wyoming	2,835,391

Source: Rea, W. 1992. Chemical Sensitivity, Vol. 2, Sources of Total Body Load. Lewis Publishers. Reprinted with permission.

Table 12.6   **Environmental Synthetic Chemicals and Thyroid**

Category	Use	Species (H,W,L)
1. Pesticides		
Amide		
Oxyacetamide (FOE 5043)	herbicide	rat
N-2-fluorenylacetamide	rodenticide	rat
Benzonitrile		
bromoxynil	herbicide	rat
ioxynil	herbicide	in vitro H
Carbamate		
carbaryl	insecticide	fish
carbofuran	insecticide	fish
Chlorophenoxy		
2,4-D	herbicide	rat
Nitrofen (diphenylether)	herbicide	mouse
Organochlorine		
aldrin insecticide		chick
alachlor	herbicide	rat
chlordane, oxy-	insecticide	rat
DDD or TDE	insecticide	rat, H
DDE	DDT metabolite	bird
DDT	insecticide	rat, bird, fish
dicofol	acaricide	in vitro
dieldrin	insecticide	rat, bird, rabbit
endosulfan	insecticide	fish
heptachlor, -epoxide	insecticide	rat
hexadrin = endrin	insecticide	fish
lindane (gBHC, gHCH)	insecticide	fish, frog, rat, rabbit, H?
mirex	insecticide	rat
pentachlorobenzene	pesticide, by-product	rat
photomirex	insecticide	rat
toxaphene	insecticide	bird, rat
trichorobenzene	herbicide, industrial	rat
Organophosphates		
dimethoate	insecticide	mice, chick
fenithrothion	insecticide	fish
malathion, cythion	insecticide	rat, fish, H
methylparathion	insecticide	rat
ronnel/fenchlorfos	insecticide	beef steers
Pyrethroid		
Karate (1-cyhalothrin)	insecticide	rat
Talstar (bifenthrin)	insecticide	rat
fenvalerate	insecticide	mouse, rat
deltamethrin	insecticide	rat
Pyridinoxy		
Picloram	herbicide	rat
Thiocarbamate		
mancozeb	fungicide	rat
maneb	fungicide	rat
nabam	fungicide	chick
zineb	fungicide	rat, rabbit

Table 12.6 cont.   **Environmental Synthetic Chemicals and Thyroid**

Category	Use	Species (H,W,L)
Thiourea		
ethylenethiourea	fungicide, rubber	rat, mice, H
Triazine		
atrazine	herbicide	rat
triazole		
aminotriazole	herbicide	rat, hamster, guinea pig, chick, H
2. Industrial chemicals		
Chlorine dioxide	disinfectant	primate, rat, pigeon
carbon disulfide	vicose	H
Heavy metal/elements		
aluminum	containers, food additives	fish
cadmium	batteries	rabbit, monkey, rat, squirrel, fish
lead	paint, pipes	H, squirrel, rat, fish, duck
mercury	thermometers, dental fillings	fish, rat, hog, rabbit, mouse
radioactive iodine	nuclear plant	H, swan
Hydroxypyridines	cigarette smoke, coal	cattle, mice, rat
Phthalates		
di2ethylhexylphthalate (DEHP)		rat, H?
di-n-hexylphthalate		rat
diisobutylphthalate		H?
di-n-octylphthalate (DnOP)		rat
diOHbenzoicacids (DHBA)	metabolite	rat
Polycyclic aromatic		
benzopyrene	smoke, combustion	rat
methylcholanthrene (MCA)	petroleum	rat
Polyhalogenated		
dioxins	byproducts	rat, mouse, hamster, H
furans	pyrolysis, by-products	monkey, H
hexachlorobenzene	fungicide	hamster, rat, H
PBB	flame retardant	bird, rat, H, sow, mouse
PCB	capacitor	H, rat, mice, monkey, bird, fish, mink, seal
polychlorinated diphenyl ether	flame retardant	rat
tetracholoro benzyltoluenes (Ugilec 141)	hydraulic fluid	mice
Polyhydroxyphenols & phenol derivatives		
dinitrophenol	insecticide, reagent	H
hydroxy(hydro)quinones	cosmetics	rat
phenol	in plywood, plastic, rubber	fish

Table 12.6 cont.   **Environmental Synthetic Chemicals and Thyroid**

Category	Use	Species (H,W,L)
pentachlorophenol	wood preservative, metabolite (HCB, pentachlorobenzene)	rat, H, cattle
resorcinol	rubber industry, coal	rat, H
Sulfurated organics	coal conversion, smoke	
thiocyanatae	coal conversion	rat, H
Vinyl acetate		rat
3. Suspected or unidentified environmental factor		H, fish, seal, phoca, duck
4. Additional chemicals[a]		bird, panther
Acetochlor	herbicide	rodent
Bromacil	herbicide	rodent
Clofentezine	miticide, acaricide	rodent
DCPA	herbicide	rodent
Ethiozin (tycor)	herbicide	rodent
Ethofenprox (trebon)	insecticide	rodent
Etridizaole	fungicide	rodent
Fenbuconazole	fungicide	rodent
Fipronil	insecticide	rodent
N-OBHD		
Pendimethalin	herbicide	rodent
Pentachloronitrobenzene	fungicide	rodent
Piperonyl butoxide	synergist	rodent
Prodiamine	herbicide	rodent
Pronamide	herbicide	rodent
Pyrethrins	insecticide	rodent
Pyrimethanil		
Terbutryn	herbicide	rodent
Thiazopyr	herbicide	rodent
Triadimefon	fungicide	rodent
Trifluralin	herbicide	rodent

L., laboratory; h, human; W, wildlife; G, goiter; TW, thyroid weight; T, tumor; K, cancer; TTR, transthyretin; Nl, normal; thyr, thyroid; BMR, basal metabolic rate; TH, thyroid hormones; DCPA, dimethyltetra-chloroterephthalate; N-OBHD, octyl bicyclohaptene dicarboximide.

Chemicals are divided into pesticides and industrial chemicals. Some compounds belong to both categories and are placed according to their main use.

aSince the time this revised paper was accepted, an important article was published (381), adding 21 more chemicals that can disrupt the thyroid function and induce thyroid tumor. This article summarizes information from EPA files, most of which are not peer reviewed papers. In the same article, another herbicide, oryzalin (class dinitroaniline), was reported to induce thyroid tumors but only at high doses.

Source: Brucker-Davis, F. 1998. Effects of Environmental Synthetic Chemicals on Thyroid Function. *Thyroid*. 8:827-856. Reprinted with permission.

Chapter 13
Treatment Results

Dr. Barnes compiled the most extensive body of research on the subject of hypothyroidism in the history of medicine. He compared the patients that he had treated with a national study called the Framingham Study. The initial Framingham Study attempted to determine the risk factors that were responsible for the massive increase in heart attacks during the twentieth century. Five thousand patients in Framingham, Massachusetts were tracked for decades, and the percentage of heart attacks occurring in separate age groups, with different risk factors such as increased cholesterol or high blood pressure, were compared. The incidence of heart attacks was determined for each group according to age, sex, and risk factors.

Dr. Barnes treated 1,569 patients during his 22 year study. Some patients participated throughout and others for the minimum requirement of two years. Treatment of 1,569 patients, for an average of five years each, resulted in nearly 9,000 years of experience with thyroid therapy. The number of heart attacks totaled four. The Framingham Study predicted 72 should have occurred. This means he prevented over 90% of the predicted heart attacks in his patients. At least 30 patients who dropped out of his study, and discontinued the use of their desiccated thyroid medication, suffered heart attacks. Dr. Barnes did not control smoking, diet, exercise, or any other factors except for their hypothyroidism. *Solved: The Riddle of Heart Attacks* was first published in 1976 and underwent eight printings. This book remains the "Rosetta Stone" of the subject of heart attacks. He provided doctors with a bibliography filled with research that supported his findings. Unfortunately, mainstream medicine apparently chose not to listen.

Around 10% of the 1,569 patients in his study had been previously diagnosed with high blood pressure. Eighty percent of these patients' blood pressure normalized after being treated with desiccated thyroid. Dr. Barnes blamed the vast majority of high blood pressure on low thyroid function. Physicians have known that high blood pressure may result from decreased blood flow to the kidneys. A hypothyroid person's circulation may be reduced by as much as 40%. Dr. Barnes believed this drop in blood flow to the kidneys to be the primary cause of high blood pressure.

The rate of patients in his study group who developed diabetes was less than 2%. America's current incidence is 6% and climbing. None of his patients with diabetes suffered any of the terrible complications that millions of diabetics and their families continue to endure. Almost all of these complications are attributable to atherosclerosis, which Dr. Barnes felt strongly could be halted in adults by taking at least two grains of desiccated thyroid.

Dr. Barnes and I came to the same conclusion regarding chronic pain and arthritis. The vast majority of chronic pain is due to hypothyroidism. Patients who were properly treated with thyroid medication but continued to suffer from arthritic pain, greatly benefited from small dosages of prednisone added to their thyroid regimen. These patients suffered none of the complications associated with the chronic use of prednisone and were relieved of the majority of their pain. In my opinion, environmentally related illnesses appear to be contributing more and more to the milieu of possible causes of pain.

About 90% of Dr. Barnes' acne patients responded to thyroid therapy. Many other skin disorders including eczema, psoriasis, boils, and impetigo, also responded to thyroid therapy.

Menstrual problems that were associated with hypothyroidism responded equally well. Over 90% of patients with painful menstruation, irregular menstrual cycles, and heavy periods returned to normal. Most of the problems associated with pregnancy were avoided altogether.

Headaches and migraines have also been symptoms associated with the hypothyroidism since The Clinical Society of London's report on myxedema in 1888. Dr. Barnes devoted a chapter to migraines and headaches in his book. Ninety-five of the first 100 patients he treated with desiccated thyroid responded well.

Dr. Sonkin blamed endocrinologists for not just missing hypothyroidism but for allowing ob-gyn doctors to dictate treatment for the menopause that conflicted with, or neglected, the mountain of literature that the New York Hospital–Cornell Medical Center had amassed during his tenure. He stated, "We dropped the ball."

Dr. Papanicolaou developed the Pap smear while working at the Endocrine Clinic of the New York Hospital–Cornell Medical Center. He and Dr. Ephraim Shorr collaborated in the development of a vaginal stain that enables doctors to precisely check an individual woman's estrogen level. I may be the only practicing physician familiar with this invaluable procedure. [Physicians interested in this procedure should know that 50% alcohol may be substituted for the highly volatile ether recommended in the initial paper.][74]

Dr. Barnes and other physicians blame a significant portion of obesity on hypothyroidism. A slow metabolism does not require many calories. Couple this with other hypothyroid symptoms such as fatigue, weakness, and you can begin to see the problem. Please read Dr. Barnes' chapter on obesity.

A host of other problems have been linked with hypothyroidism. In Dr. Barnes' opinion, 99 times out of 100, when a low basal temperature is associated with an illness, a trial of thyroid medication is called for. I agree completely.

Lack of Acceptance

The lack of acceptance I encounter, and people's unwillingness to explore the literature, is disappointing. People rarely like being told that they have hypothyroidism or adrenal deficiency. The thought of being dependent upon medication for the remainder of their lives is unsettling. However, these same patients have no qualms about taking multiple prescriptions for depression, diabetes, high blood pressure, high cholesterol, anxiety, insomnia, recurrent infections, chronic pain, and other conditions that result from hypothyroidism. Many patients are grateful to have a logical explanation and treatment for their suffering.

Initially, patients rarely asked to have their children treated. Many may not want to accept the fact that they have passed on deleterious genes and toxins to their offspring. One of my patient's responses upon being told her granddaughter needed treatment was, "How could there possibly be anything wrong with that beautiful child." The child was seeing an orthopedist for pain and was very short for her age.

The overwhelming majority of primary care doctors caution patients to beware of my recommendations no matter how severely the patients are suffering. The standard thyroid blood test results are usually in the "normal range".

The problems of acceptance among patients that I encountered in Columbia, Missouri are less problematic in Paradise Valley, Arizona. There is a large population of enlightened alternative care practitioners who are aware of the Barnes Foundation, mild adrenal deficiencies, Candidiasis, heavy metal toxicity, and environmental toxins. Many current patients were apprised of their problems by their chiropractors or other alternative caregivers before being referred to me. Currently, medical doctors are the only ones capable of prescribing the necessary hormones or administering a number of other important interventions.

The International Society for Orthomolecular Medicine's aim is to restore the optimum environment of the body by correcting imbalances or deficiencies based on individual biochemistry using substances such as vitamins, minerals, amino acids, trace elements, and essential fatty acids. Many of these doctors are proficient in the usage of desiccated thyroid and bio-identical hormones such as estrogen, progesterone, and testosterone. These doctors are adept at treating mental illnesses including schizophrenia.

416 733-2117 (Toronto, Canada)
www.orthomed.org

Chapter 14
Conclusion

Modern science has recognized the importance of inheritance in a large percentage of our chronic illnesses such as cancer, diabetes, mental illness, high blood pressure, heart disease, and arthritis.

Current texts, regarding the thyroid and its diseases, include chapters on genetically inherited hypothyroidism, but continue to insist the occurrence is rare. Drs. Barnes and Sonkin believed inherited problems, particularly at the cellular level, were responsible for the epidemic of hypothyroidism. Defective mitochondria, our chemical energy factories that are inherited solely from the mother, appear to be the most likely culprits. Environmental toxins greatly exacerbate and accelerate the epidemic.

Medicine has become so technologically advanced and specialized that doctors and scientists are unable to see the forest for the trees. Blood tests do not reveal the inherited or environmentally related forms of Type 2 hypothyroidism. Full-blown cases of hypothyroidism present themselves regularly in doctors' offices and go unnoticed.

Basal temperature, basal metabolism, pathology and autopsy studies, and long-term treatment results on thousands of patients were completed decades ago as mentioned in this text.

Long-term medical observations on groups of patients have been shown to be as efficacious as double-blind studies. Dr. Barnes' thyroid study lasted well over 20 years and involved over 1,500 patients. No other study in the history of medicine offered as much promise. Double-blind studies were not necessary for the polio vaccine or for penicillin. Our populace is suffering greatly and need not be subjected to more testing, because the answers are available.[27]

A fundamental shift away from the current medical dogma on hypothyroidism will be required in order for the populace to receive the help that they so desperately need.

For those who doubt the validity of my presentation, please do what I did. Read Dr. Barnes' books and the papers listed in his bibliographies, as well as in mine. Study the works of Dr. Zondek, Dr. Sonkin, and the Doctors Hertoghe (all four generations of them). You will find a mountain of literature and clinical evidence by prominent doctors and scientists that has been forgotten or ignored. If you choose to dismiss this work, the result will be a continued increase in the current epidemic of chronic illness and suffering.

Autopsy and pathology studies extricated us from the abyss of medieval medicine. A similar scenario will be necessary to remove any doubts regarding the pervasiveness of Type 2 hypothyroidism. The abnormal accumulation of mucin in our connective tissue is unique to hypothyroidism. Biopsies from living patients and those from autopsies were formerly used to confirm the diagnosis. I asked a senior pathologist when he last performed a biopsy looking for hypothyroidism. His answer was the one I expected, "Never".

Any doubt about the pervasiveness of Type 2 hypothyroidism would be quickly settled if autopsies were performed on the next 100 obese patients who suffered an early death from heart attack. Taking a tiny section of the parotid gland during the autopsy and using the Periodic acid-Schiff (PAS) stain to demonstrate the presence of mucin in the parotid gland would clearly prove that hypothyroidism is the underlying cause of death. If someone in your family falls into this category, you might want to ask for this test to be done at the autopsy. The test result could have a significant impact on how you view the health status of the remaining members of your family.

Now that you understand that you or someone in your family may have Type 2 hypothyroidism, you can seek out the needed help. There are doctors around the world that know and understand how to treat this disease. By knowing what to look for and how to treat it, you can find a doctor and work with them to effect a change.

For additional information visit my Website at:

www.type2hypothyroidism.com

Appendix A
Physiologic Functions of the Thyroid Hormones

Source: Guyton, A. *Textbook of Medical Physiology*. Philadelphia: WB Saunders Company, 2000. Reprinted with permission from Elsevier.

Thyroid Hormones Increase the Transcription of Large Numbers of Genes

The general effect of thyroid hormone is to activate nuclear transcription of large numbers of genes. Therefore, in virtually all cells of the body, great numbers of proteins, and other substances are synthesized. The net result is generalized increase in functional activity throughout the body.

Most of the thyroxine secreted by the thyroid is converted to triiodothyronine. Before acting on the genes to increase genetic transcription, one iodide is removed from almost all the thyroxine, thus forming triiodothyronine. Intracellular thyroid hormone receptors have a very high affinity for triiodothyronine. Consequently, about 90% of the thyroid hormone molecules that bind with the receptors is triiodothyronine and only 10% thyroxine.

Thyroid hormones activate nuclear receptors. The thyroid receptors are either attached to the DNA genetic strands or located in proximity to them. On binding with thyroid hormone, the receptors become activated and initiate the transcription process. Then large numbers of different types of messenger RNA are formed, followed within another few minutes or hours by RNA translation on the cytoplasmic ribosomes to form hundreds of new intracellular proteins. However, not all the proteins are increased by similar percentages—some only slightly and others at least as much as six-fold. It is believed that most, if not all, of the actions of thyroid hormone result from the subsequent enzymatic and other functions of these new proteins.

Thyroid Hormones Increase Cellular Metabolic Activity

The thyroid hormones increase the metabolic activities of almost all the tissues of the body. The basal metabolic rate can increase from 60% to 100% above normal when large quantities of the hormones are secreted. The rate of utilization of foods for energy is greatly accelerated. Although the rate of protein synthesis is increased, at the same time the rate of protein catabolism is also increased. The growth rate of young people is greatly accelerated. The mental processes are excited, and the activities of most of the other endocrine glands are increased.

Thyroid hormones increase the number and activity of mitochondria. When thyroxine or triiodothyronine is given to an animal, the mitochondria in most cells of the animal's body increase in size as well as number. Furthermore, the total membrane surface area of the mitochondria increases almost directly in proportion to the increased metabolic rate of the whole animal. Therefore, one of principle functions of thyroxine might be simply to increase the number and activity of mitochondria, which in turn increases the rate of formation of adenosine triphosphate (ATP) to energize cellular function. However, the increase in the number and activity of mitochondria could be the result of increased activity of the cells, as well as the cause of the increase.

Thyroid hormones increase active transport of ions through cell membranes. One of the enzymes that becomes increased in response to thyroid hormone is Na, K-ATPase. This in turn increases the rate of transport of both sodium and potassium ions through the cell membranes of some tissue. Because this process uses energy and increases the amount of heat produced in the body, it has been suggested that this might be one of the mechanisms by which thyroid hormone increases the body's metabolic rate. In fact, thyroid hormone also causes the cell membranes of most cells to become leaky to sodium ions, which further activates the sodium pump and further increases heat production.

Effect of Thyroid Hormone on Growth

Thyroid hormone has both general and specific effects on growth. For instance, it has long been known that thyroid hormone is essential for the metamorphic change of the tadpole into the frog.

In humans, the effect of thyroid hormone on growth is manifest mainly in growing children. In those who are hypothyroid, the rate of growth is greatly retarded. In those who are hypothyroid, excessive skeletal growth often occurs, causing the child to become considerably taller at an earlier age. However, the bones also mature more rapidly and the epiphyses close at an early age, so that the duration of growth and the eventual height of the adult may actually be shortened.

An important effect of thyroid hormone is to promote growth and development of the brain during fetal life and for the first few years of postnatal life. If the fetus does not secrete sufficient quantities of thyroid hormone, growth and maturation of the brain both before birth and afterward are greatly retarded, and the brain remains smaller than normal. Without specific thyroid therapy within days or weeks after birth the child without a thyroid gland will remain mentally deficient throughout life.

Effect of Thyroid Hormone on Specific Bodily Mechanisms

Stimulation of Carbohydrates Metabolism. Thyroid hormone stimulates almost all aspects of carbohydrate metabolism, including rapid uptake of glucose by the cells, enhanced glycolysis, enhanced gluconeogenesis, increased rate of absorption from the gastrointestinal tract, and even increased insulin secretion with its resultant secondary effects on carbohydrate metabolism. All these effects probably result from the overall increase in cellular metabolic enzymes caused by thyroid hormone.

Stimulation of Fat Metabolism. Essentially all aspects of fat metabolism are also enhanced under the influence of thyroid hormone. In particular, lipids are mobilized rapidly from the fat tissue, which decreases the fat stores of the body to a greater extent than almost any other tissue element. This also increases the free fatty acid concentration in the plasma and greatly accelerates the oxidation of free fatty acids by the cells.

Effect on plasma and liver fats. Increased thyroid hormone decreases the concentrations of cholesterol, phospholipids, and triglycerides in the plasma, even though it increases the free fatty acids. Conversely, decreased thyroid secretion greatly increases the plasma concentrations of cholesterol, phospholipids, and triglycerides and almost always causes excessive deposition of fat in the liver as well. The large increase in circulation plasma cholesterol in prolonged hypothyroidism is often associated with severe arteriosclerosis.

One of the mechanisms by which thyroid hormone decreases the plasma cholesterol concentration is to increase significantly the rate of cholesterol secretion in the bile and consequent loss in the feces. A possible mechanism for the increased cholesterol secretion is that thyroid hormone induces increased numbers of low-density lipoprotein receptors on the liver cells, leading to rapid removal of low-density lipoproteins from the plasma by the liver and subsequent secretion of cholesterol in these lipoproteins by the liver cells.

Increased Requirement for Vitamins. Because thyroid hormone increases the quantities of many bodily enzymes and because vitamins are essential parts of some of the enzymes or coenzymes, thyroid hormone causes increased need for vitamins. Therefore, a relative vitamin deficiency can occur when excess thyroid hormone is secreted, unless at the same time increased quantities of vitamins are made available.

Increased Basal Metabolic Rate. Because thyroid hormone increases metabolism in almost all cells of the body, excessive quantities of the hormone can occasionally increase the basal metabolic rate from 60% to 100% above normal. Conversely, when no thyroid hormone is produced, the basal metabolic rate falls to almost one-half normal.

Extreme amounts of the hormones are required to cause very high basal metabolic rates.

Decreased Body Weight. Greatly increased thyroid hormone almost always decreases the body weight, and greatly decreased hormone almost always increases body weight; these effects do not always occur, because thyroid hormone also increases the appetite, and this may counterbalance the change in the metabolic rate.

Effect of Thyroid Hormones on the Cardiovascular System

Increased Blood Flow and Cardiac Output. Increased metabolism in the tissues causes more rapid utilization of oxygen than normal and release of greater than normal quantities of metabolic end products from the tissues. These effects cause vasodilatation in most body tissues, thus increasing blood flow in the skin because of the increased need for heat elimination from the body.

As a consequence of the increased blood flow, cardiac output also increases, sometimes rising to 60% or more above normal when excessive thyroid hormone is present and falling to only 50% of normal in very severe hypothyroidism.

Increased Heart Rate. The heart rate increases considerably more under the influence of thyroid hormone than would be expected from the increase in cardiac output. Therefore, thyroid hormone seems to have a direct effect on the excitability of the heart, which in turn increases the heart rate. This rate is one of the sensitive physical signs that the clinician uses in determining whether a patient has excessive or diminished thyroid hormone production.

Increased Heart Strength. The increased enzymatic activity caused by thyroid hormone production apparently increases the strength of the heart when only a slight excess of thyroid hormone is secreted. This is analogous to the marked increase in the heart muscle strength that occurs in mild fevers and during exercise. However, when thyroid hormone is increased markedly, the heart muscle strength becomes depressed because of long-term excessive protein catabolism. Indeed, some severely thyro-toxic patients die of cardiac decompensation secondary to myocardial failure and to increased cardiac load imposed by the increase in cardiac output.

Normal Arterial Pressure. The mean arterial pressure usually remains about normal after administration of thyroid hormone. However, because of increased blood flow through the tissues between heartbeats, the pulse pressure is often increased, with the systolic pressure elevated in hyperthyroidism 10 to 15 mm Hg and the diastolic pressure reduced a corresponding amount.

Increased Respiration. The increased rate of metabolism increases the utilization of oxygen and formation of carbon dioxide; these effects activate all the mechanisms that increase the rate and depth of respiration.

Increased Gastrointestinal Motility. In addition to increased appetite and food intake, which had been discussed, thyroid hormone increases both the rates of secretion of the digestive juices and the motility of the gastrointestinal tract. Diarrhea often results from <u>hyper</u>thyroidism. Lack of thyroid hormone can cause constipation.

Excitatory Effects on the Central Nervous System. In general, thyroid hormone increases the rapidity of cerebration but also often dissociates this; conversely, lack of thyroid hormone decreases this function. The <u>hyper</u>thyroid individual is likely to have extreme nervousness and many psychoneurotic tendencies, such as anxiety complexes, extreme worry, and paranoia.

Effect on the Function of the Muscles. Slight increase in thyroid hormone usually makes the muscles react with vigor, but when the quantity of hormone becomes excessive, the muscles become weakened because of excess protein catabolism. Conversely, lack of thyroid hormone causes the muscles to become sluggish, and they relax slowly after contraction.

Muscle Tremor. One of the most characteristic signs of <u>hyper</u>thyroidism is a fine muscle tremor. This is not the coarse tremor that occurs in Parkinson's disease or in shivering, because it occurs at the rapid frequency of 10 to 15 times per second. The tremor can be observed easily by placing a sheet of paper on the extended fingers and noting the degree of vibration of the paper. This tremor is believed to be caused by increased reactivity of the neuronal synapses in the areas of the spinal cord that control muscle tone. The tremor is an important means for assessing the degree of thyroid hormone effect on the central nervous system.

Effect on Sleep. Because of the exhausting effect of thyroid hormone on the musculature and on the central nervous system, the <u>hyper</u>thyroid subject often has a feeling of constant tiredness; but because of the excitable effects of thyroid hormone on the synapses, it is difficult to sleep. Conversely, extreme somnolence is characteristic of hypothyroidism, with sleep sometimes lasting 12 to 14 hours a day.

Effect on Other Endocrine Glands. Increased thyroid hormone increases the rates of secretion of most other endocrine glands, but it also increases the need of the tissues for the hormones. For instance, increased thyroxine secretion increases the rate of glucose metabolism everywhere in the body, and therefore, causes a corresponding need for increased insulin secretion by the pancreas. Also, thyroid hormone increases many metabolic activities related to bone formation and, as a consequence, increases the need for parathyroid hormone. Finally, thyroid hormone increases the rate at which adrenal glucocorticoid secretes by the adrenal glands.

Effect of Thyroid Hormone on Sexual Function. For normal sexual function, thyroid secretion needs to be approximately normal. In men, lack of thyroid hormone is likely to cause loss of libido; whereas great excesses of the hormone sometimes cause impotence. A hypothyroid woman, like a man, is likely to have greatly decreased libido.

In women, lack of thyroid hormone often causes menorrhagia and polymenorrhea, that is respectively, excessive and frequent menstrual bleeding. Yet, strangely enough, in other women thyroid lack may cause irregular periods and occasionally even amenorrhea.

To make the picture still more confusing, in the hyperthyroid woman, oligomenorrhea, which means "greatly reduced bleeding," is common, and occasionally amenorrhea results.

The action of thyroid hormone on the gonads cannot be pinpointed to a specific function but probably results from a combination of direct metabolic effects on the gonads, as well as excitatory and inhibitory feedback effects operating through the anterior pituitary hormones that control the sexual functions.

Appendix B
Mechanisms of Thyroid Hormone Disruption by Synthetic Chemicals

There are many steps in the chemical reactions required to properly utilize thyroid hormones. The following chart is an overview of these different steps and the synthetic chemicals that disrupt them.

See Table B.1 on next page.

Table B.1

Synthetic Chemicals that Interfere with the Production, Transport, and Metabolism of Thyroid Hormone.

Thyroid mechanism and interfering chemical

Uptake of iodide by thyroid gland
2,4-D (137)
3-Amino-1,2,4-triazole (138,139)
Aldrin(140)
Amitrole (141, 142)
Aroclor (141, 142)
1,2-Dihydroxybenzene (catechol)(146)
4-Chlororesorcinol (146)
Clofentezine (141)
o-Cresol (146)
p-Cresol (146)
Cythion (96, 147)
1,3-Dihydroxynaphthalene (146)
1,5-Dihydroxynaphthalene (146)
2,3-Dihydroxynaphthalene (146)
2,7-Dihydroxynaphthalene (146)
2,4-Dihydroxybenzaldehyde (146)
2,4-Dihydroxybenzoic acid (146)
Ethiozin (141)
Ethylene thiourea (141, 148)
Fipronil (141)
Hexachlorobenzene(149,150)
Hexadrin (147)
4-Hexylresorcinol (146)
1,3,4-Trihydroxybenzene (hydroxyquinol) (146)
Hydroxyquinol triacetate(146)
Lead (151)
Mancozeb (152)
Mercuric chloride (153,154)
3-Methylcholanthrene (143, 155)
Methylmercuric chloride (154)
Methylaparthion (156)
2-Methylresorcinol (146)
Mull-Soy (157)
Nabam (140)
5-Methylresorcinol (orcinol) (146)
Pendimethalin (141)
Pentachloronitrobenzene (141)
Phenobarbital (143)
Phenol (146)
1,3,5-Trihydroxybeozene (phloroglucinol) (146)
Polybrominated biphenyls (158)
Pregnenolone-16α-carbonitrile (143)
Propylthiouracil (139, 158)
1,2,3-Trihydroxybenzene pyrogallol) (146)
Pyrimentanil (141)
1,3-Dihyroxybenzene(resorcinol) (146)
o-Hydroxybenzyl alcohol (saligenin) (146)
Selenium (151)
Thiocyanate (141)

Sodium/iodide symporter
Perchlorate (94, 159)
Perrhenate (159)

Serum protein-bound iodide level
2,4-D (137)
2,4-Dinitrophenol (96)
3-Methylcholanthrene (155)
Amitrole (142)
Aroclor 1254 (144)
Cythion (95, 147)
Malathion (160)
Mancozeb (152)
Mercuric chloride (153)

o,p'-DDD (161,162)
Hexadrin (147)

Thyroid peroxidase action—general information
Amitrole (141)
Ammonia (154)
Ethylene thiouree (141)
Fipronil (141)
Mancozeb (141)
4,4'-Methylenedianiline (141)
Thiocyante (141)

Thyroid peroxidase action—oxidation of iodide
Aminotriazole (97, 164)
Ammonia (163)
Cadmium chloride (163, 165)
Endosulfan (166)
Ethylene thiourea (98)
1,2,3,4,5,6-Hexachlorocyclohexane (lindane) (167)
Malathion (167)
Mancozeb (152)
Mercury chloride (165)
Methamizole (97)
Polybrominated biphenyls (158)
Thiourea (166)

Thyroid peroxidase action—iodination of tyrosine
Polybrominated biphenyls (158)

Binding to thyroglobulin
o,p'-DDD (161)
Pentachlorophenol (168)

Binding to transthyretin
Bromoxynil (3.5-bibromo-4-hydroxybenzonitril) (99)
4-(Chloro-o-tolyloxy) acetic acid (99)
4-(4-Chloro-2-methylphenoxy) butyric acid (99)
Chlorophenol (99, 169)
Chloroxuron (99)
2,4-D (99)
2,4-Dicholorophenoxybutric acid (99)
Dioxtylpthalete (99)
o,p'-DDD (99)
p,p'-DDD(99)
2,3-Dichlorophenol (99, 169)
2,4-Dichlorophenol (99)
2,6-Dichlorophenol (99, 169, 170)
2-(2.4-Dicholorophenoxy) propionic acid [dichloroprop] (99)
1,1,1-Trichloro-2,2-bis(chlorophenol) ethanol [difocol] (99)
2,4-Dinitrophenol (99)
2,4-Dinitro-6-methyphenol (99)
Ethyl-bromophos (99)
Ethyl-parathion (99)
2-(2,4,5-Trichlorophenoxy) propionic acid [fenoprop] (99)
Hexachlorobenzene (99)
Hexachlorophene (99, 169)
2-Hydroxybiphenyl (99)
4-Hydroxybiphenyl (99, 169)
Lindane (99)
Linuron (99)
Malathion (99)
Pentachlorophenol (99, 169, 170)
Phenol (169)

Pyrogallol (99)
2,4,5-Trichlorophenoxyacetic acid (99)
1,4-Tetrachlorophenol (99, 170)
PCB-77 (99, 105, 169)
Trichloroacetic acid (99)
2,3,4-Trichlorophenol (170)
2,4,5-Trichlorophenol (99, 169, 170)
2,4,6-Trichlorophenol (99, 170)
2,4,5-Trichlorophenoxyacetic acid methyl ester (99)

Binding to albumin
Pentachlorophenol (169)

Catabolism of T4 or T3: type I or II 5'-deiodinase
3,3',4,4',5,5'-Hexachlorobiphenyl (107)
3-Methylcholanthrene (171, 172)
Aminotriazole (106)
Amiodarone (94, 172)
Aroclor 1254 (109)
Cadmium chloride (173)
Diphrmylthiohydantoin (141,172)
Dimethoate (100, 174)
Fenvalerate (175,176)
Hexachlorobenzene (102)
Lead (177)
Phenobarbital (172)
Propylthiouracil (172)
PCB 77 (107, 171)
TCDD (171, 178)

Glucuronidation of T4/T3
Acetochlor (141)
Aroclor 1254 (109, 143-145, 179)
3,4-Benzpyrene (180)
Clofentenzine (141)
Clofibrate (141)
DDT (144)
Fenbuconazole (141)
3,3',4,4',5,5'-Hexabromobiphenyl (101)
Hexachlorobenzene (102, 183)
2,3,3',4,4',5-Hexachlorobiphenyl (182)
3,3',4,4',5,5'-Hexachlorobiphenyl (107)
3-Methylcholanthrene (141, 143, 155, 171, 179)
Pendimethalin (141)
PCB 126 (108, 182)
Phenobarbital (141, 143, 172, 180, 181, 183)
Polybrominated biphenyls (184)
PCBs (141)
Pregnenolone-16α-carbonitrile (141, 143, 179)
Promadiamine (141)
Pyrimethanil (141)
PCB 77 (108, 171)
TCDD (108, 141, 178, 182)
Thiazopyr (141)

Catabolism and biliary elimination of T4/ T3 in the liver
Aroclor 1254 (144, 145)
3,4-Benzopyrene (180)
DDT (144)
Hexachlorobenzene (102)
3-Methylcholanthrene (155)
Phenobabital (180, 183)
Polybrominated biphenyls (184)

Abbreviations: 2,4-D 2,4-dichlorophenoxyacetic acid; DDD 1-1dichloro-2, 2-histo-chlorophenyllethane.

Source: Howdeshell, K. A Model of the Development of the Brain as a Construct of the Thyroid System. *Environmental Health Perspectives* 2002; 110(supp 3):337-8.

Appendix C
Appeal for Contributions to Protect Patient Rights
For Treatment for Environmental Injuries

Dear Friends,

I am reaching out to you today asking for your support of Dr. William Rea and for the future of the Environmental Health Center – Dallas. Perhaps at EHC-D you have learned about your health and your environment, perhaps you have recovered quality to your life or perhaps, like me, you have received life-saving treatment from the devastating effects of severe chemical injury. Many, many of us, in fact thousands of people from around the world who suffer from chemical injury and environmental sensitivity have found a refuge of understanding, appropriate and effective medical treatment and a return to functionality and good health, solely through the innovative knowledge and medical care of Dr. Rea.

Friends, the time is now to offer your support for Dr. Rea, this pioneering physician of environmental medicine and provider of a 30 year foundation of knowledge for which the treatment of chemical injury and sensitivity is built. For the past three years, the Texas Medical Board, acting under pressure from insurance companies, is trying to disallow the practice of environmental medicine by relentlessly attacking the integrity and professional knowledge of Dr. Rea and now that of many other physicians who also offer environmental medical treatment. This is an exhaustive and costly endeavor for Dr. Rea to continue championing your right for access to appropriate and effective treatment for chemical sensitivity and injury. A legal defense fund is being created to sustain Dr. Rea's legal representation and to help insure that environmental medicine has the respected and enduring future that it rightly deserves.

You can contribute your donation to the:

Attention: Ellie
William J. Rea Legal Defense Fund"
8345 Walnut Hill Lane - Suite 220
Dallas, Texas 75231

Your effort to help Dr. Rea is both meaningful and needed, no matter how small or how large your contribution may be. The entire amount of your donation will be used exclusively for Dr. Rea's legal defense. This letter comes to you with the full endorsement of Dr. Rea and is an official communication of the Environmental Health Center–Dallas. Thank you for your generous support of Dr. Rea and for your unity in the preservation of environmental medicine.

With Warm Regards,

Barbra Pond

Source: Environmental Health Center–Dallas Staff/Author EHC-D Newsletter

Glossary

Arteriosclerosis: a chronic disease that impairs blood flow by thickening, hardening, or loss of elasticity of the arterial walls.

Atherosclerosis: clogging, narrowing, and hardening of the large and medium sized arteries, which can cause heart attack, stroke, kidney and eye problems.

Autosome: any paired chromosome in males and females that is not a sex chromosome; humans have 22 pairs plus the 2 sex chromosomes (XX= female, XY= male) for a total of 46 chromosomes.

Autosomal dominant: a dominant or controlling genetic influence capable of expression (the trait is manifested) when carried by only one of the two paired autosomes; the physical trait is expressed if a dominant gene is carried by either parent.

Autosomal recessive: both chromosomes of a pair of autosomes must carry the same genetic trait (gene) in order for it to be expressed.

Basal metabolism: the minimal energy expended for the main-tenance of respiration, circulation, body temperature, glandular activity, muscle tone, and the other basic functions of the body.

Basal temperature: the temperature of the body under conditions of absolute rest.

Chromosomes: a structure in the nucleus containing a linear thread of DNA, which transmits genetic information during cell division; 46 are normally present in man.

Claw toes: deformity of the toes where the proximal joints are hyperextended (bent upwards) and the distal joints are flexed (bent downwards) producing a claw-like appearance.

Congenital: conditions that are present at birth (usually before birth).

Connective tissue: the tissue that binds together and is the support of the various structures of the body.

Cretin: a person affected with cretinism.

Cretinism: arrested physical and mental development due to a congenital lack of thyroid hormone secretion. This condition also results from congenital Type 2 hypothyroidism in varying degrees of severity. Myxedema (hypothyroidism) is the acquired form of the same illness that begins after birth.

Deiodination: the loss or removal of iodine from a compound.

Eclampsia: convulsions and coma occurring during a pregnancy or following delivery; also associated with high blood pressure, edema, and proteinuria (protein in urine due to compromised function of the kidneys).

Electrocardiogram: a graphic tracing of the variations in electrical potential caused by the excitation of the heart muscle and detected at the body surface; also known as ECG or EKG.

Electroencephalogram: a recording of the electrical potentials on the skull that are generated by electrical currents emanating from the nerve cells in the brain.

Enzymes: a protein molecule that catalyzes chemical reactions of other substances without itself being destroyed or altered upon completion of the reactions.

Fibromyalgia: widespread chronic pain and stiffness in the muscles, tendons, and ligaments (soft tissues) that is usually associated with weakness and fatigue; women are affected more often than men.

Formication: abnormal sensations as if ants are crawling around on the skin.

Free radicals: unstable atoms or groups of atoms with an odd number of (unpaired) electrons that are able to attack other molecules or important cellular components; antioxidants such as vitamin C can neutralize free radicals.

Galactorrhea: excessive or spontaneous flow of milk, or persistent secretion of milk irrespective of nursing.

Gene: a segment of a DNA molecule that contains all of the information required for synthesis of a product.

Goiter: an enlargement of the thyroid gland that is not associated with inflammation or cancer.

Hyperthyroidism: excessive functioning of the thyroid gland with increased secretion of thyroid hormones. Symptoms may include a rapid heartbeat, atrial fibrillation, weight loss, muscular weakness, nervousness, tremor, heat intolerance, bulging eyes, and frequent bowel movements.

Hypoglycemia: an abnormally low concentration of sugar (glucose) in the blood, which may lead to headache, irritability, cold sweats, shakiness, tremors, bizarre behavior, and ultimately convulsions and coma in severe cases.

Hypothyroidism: deficiency of thyroid activity that is marked by lowered basal metabolism, subnormal body temperature, and myxedema. Also see Type 1 hypothyroidism and Type 2 hypothyroidism.

Jaundice: a yellow color in the skin, mucous membranes, and the eyes due to excess bilirubin. Bilirubin is formed mostly from a breakdown product of red blood cells.

Mania: mood disorder marked by agitation, hyperexcitability, increased speed of thought and speech, and elation.

Meniere's disease: a syndrome marked by hearing loss, tinnitus (noises or ringing in the ears), and vertigo due to an inner ear disorder (distention of the membranous labyrinth); named after French physician, Prosper Meniere (1799-1862).

Metabolism: the sum of all the physical and chemical processes by which living organized substance is produced and maintained, and also the transformation by which energy is made available for use by the organism.

Mitochondria: small organelles that are the principle sites of the body's energy production; they contain DNA and RNA and can independently replicate and code for the synthesis of some of their proteins.

Morphology: the form and structure of a particular organism, or the science of the forms and structure of organisms.

Mucin: a nitrogenous glue-like substance found in all the secretions of mucous glands and also between the fibers of connective tissues; an abnormally large accumulation of mucin is the hallmark of hypothyroidism (myxedema).

Myxedema: the medical term for hypothyroidism; named for the abnormal accumulation of mucin (myx = Greek for mucin) and the characteristic firm edema (swelling) that results from the accumulation of mucin.

Neurosis: a functional mental disorder such as obsessions, anxiety attacks, and phobias; sufferers are usually aware of their neurosis and reality testing is intact (as compared to psychosis where reality testing is impaired).

Nucleus: the central part of a living cell containing chromosomes and other genetic information.

Orthotic: an orthopedic device intended to improve or restore the function of the movable body parts.

Parotid gland: largest of the human salivary glands.

Pathognomonic: a characteristic symptom or sign of an illness or disease that allows a definitive diagnosis to be made.

Peripheral resistance syndrome: peripheral cellular resistance or inadequate cellular response to normal levels of thyroid hormones in the blood; a form of Type 2 hypothyroidism.

Physiognomy: judging the character of something by its outward appearance, usually pertaining to the face.

Pituitary gland: one of the primary endocrine glands in vertebrates that secretes a variety of critical hormones including the thyroid stimulating hormone (TSH).

Porcine: pertaining to or derived from pigs.

Precocious: more developed or advanced than usual for a particular age; or excessive development.

Scoliosis: abnormal lateral curvature of the spine.

Symptomatic low metabolism: syndrome pertaining to peripheral resistance to normal blood levels of thyroid hormones, a form of Type 2 hypothyroidism.

Tender points: exquisitely tender small knots in muscles, ligaments, or fascia (fascia is the connective tissue that covers muscles, tendons, and binds together other body parts).

Thyroprival: pertaining to hypothyroidism.

Thyroid: pertaining to the thyroid gland; also used in reference to desiccated thyroid from porcine thyroid glands.

Tinnitus: a chronic condition marked by ringing or roaring sounds in the ears.

Trigger points: tender points or knots in muscles, ligaments, or fascia that refer pain or abnormal sensations to another area of the body.

TSH: thyroid stimulating hormone produced by the pituitary gland to stimulate synthesis of more thyroid hormones.

Type 1 hypothyroidism: failure of the thyroid gland to produce sufficient amounts of thyroid hormones necessary to maintain "normal" blood levels of the thyroid stimulating hormone (TSH) produced by the pituitary gland.

Type 2 hypothyroidism: peripheral resistance to thyroid hormones at the cellular level. It is not due to a lack of thyroid hormones. Normal amounts of thyroid hormones and thyroid stimulating hormone (TSH) are usually detected by blood tests. Type 2 hypothyroidism is usually inherited. However, environmental toxins may also cause or exacerbate the problem.

Tyrosine: an amino acid that is necessary for the production (a precursor) of thyroid hormones.

Vitiligo: a medical condition resulting in smooth depigmented white patches on the skin, usually involving the face, hands, and feet.

Xanthoma: a yellowish skin lesion or tumor filled with fat (lipid), often located on the eyelids, usually due to a disorder of fat metabolism.

i

References

1   Report of a Committee of The Clinical Society of London to Investigate the Subject of Myxedema. Transactions Clinical Society London 1888; Vol. 21(suppl).

2   Hertoghe E. *The Practitioner.* Jan 1915; Vol XCIV, No. 1, 26-69.

3   Anderson H, Asboe-Hansen G, Quaade F. Histopathologic examination of the skin in the diagnosis of myxedema in children. *Journal Clinical Endocrinology.* 1955; 15:459.

4   Barnes B, Galton L. *Hypothyroidism: The Unsuspected Illness.* New York: Harper and Row Publishers; 1976.

5   Rachlin ES. *Myofascial Pain and Fibromyalgia.* St. Louis: Mosby; 1994.

6   Gelb H. *Clinical Management of Head, Neck, and TMJ Pain and Dysfunction.* Philadelphia: WB Saunders; 1977.

7   Allbutt TC. *A System of Medicine.* London: Macmillan and Company; 1901. Pages 469-484.

8   Zondek H. *Diseases of the Endocrine Glands.* 4th ed. Baltimore: The Williams & Wilkins Company; 1944.

9   Barnes BO. Basal temperature versus basal metabolism. *Journal of American Medical Association.* 1942; 119:1072-3.

10 Barnes BO. *Thyroid Therapy I, II, III* (Audio Tapes) Copies available through The Broda O. Barnes M.D. Research Foundation (www.brodabarnes.org).

11 Braverman LE, Utiger RD, Utiger RD, Ingbar SH, Werner SC. eds. *Warner & Ingbar's The Thyroid: A Fundamental and Clinical Text.* 8th ed. Philadelphia: Lippincott, Williams & Wilkins Publishers; 2000.

12 Kraus H, Hirschland B. Minimum fitness of school children. *Res Q.* 1954; 25(2):178-188.

13 Boyle R. The report that shocked the President. *Sports Illustrated.* July 1955.

14 Kraus H, Marcus NJ. Technological advance amidst humanistic decline: Ignoring muscle evaluation and treatment in the modern age of medicine. *Journal of Back and Musculoskeletal Rehabilitation.* 1997; 8(2):83-85.

15 Hill RB, Anderson RE. The recent history of the autopsy. *Archives Pathology Lab Med: Historical Perspective.* 1996; 120:702-712.

16 McPhee S. The autopsy: An antidote to misdiagnosis. *Medicine.* 1996; 75(1):41-43.

17   Ross R. Mechanisms of Disease—Atherosclerosis—An inflammatory disease. *New England Journal of Medicine*. 1999; 340(2):115-123.

18   Strong JP, McGill HC. The pediatric aspects of atherosclerosis. *Journal Atherosclerosis Research*. 1969; 9:251.

19   Ord WM. On myoxoedema, a term proposed to be applied to an essential condition in the cretinoid infection occasionally observed in middle- aged women. *Trans Med-Churg Society London*. 1877-1878; 60-1:57-78.

20   Barnes BO., Ratzenhofer M, Gisi R. The role of natural consequences in the changing death patterns. *Journal American of the American Geriatrics Society*. 1974; 22:176.

21   Campbell RE., Hughes FA. The development of bronchogenic carcinoma in patients with pulmonary tuberculosis. *J Thorac Cardiovasc Surgery*. 1960; 40:89-101.

22   Barnes BO. *Heart Attack Rareness in Thyroid-Treated Patients*. Springfield, IL: Charles C. Thomas. 1972.

23   Barnes BO. *Solved: The Riddle of Heart Attacks*. Trumbull, CT: The Broda O. Barnes M.D. Research Foundation. 1976.

24   Congress of the European Society of Cardiology, Stockholm Sweden. January 2002.

25   Espinola-Klein C, Rupprecht HJ, Blankenberg S, Bickel C, Kopp H, Rippin G, et al. Impact of infectious burden on extent and long-term prognosis of atherosclerosis. *Circulation*. 2002; 105(1):15-21.

26   Braunwald E. Shattuck lecture—cardiovascular medicine at the turn of the millennium: Triumphs, concerns and opportunities. *New England Journal of Medicine*. 1997; 337(19):1360-1369.

27   Hartz A, Benson KA. Comparison of observational studies and randomized, controlled trials. *New England Journal of Medicine*. 2000; 342:1878-86.

28   Barnes BO. On the genesis of atherosclerosis. *Journal of the American Geriatrics Society*. 1973; 21(8):350-354.

29   Mazel MS. A surgeon reviews a half century of progress in the treatment of coronary heart disease. *Journal of the American Geriatrics Society*. 1973; 21(8):355.

30   Eaton CD. Co-existence of hypothyroidism with diabetes mellitus. *Journal Michigan Medical Society*. 1954; 53:1101.

31   Zondek H. The myxedema heart. *Munchen Medical WSCHR*. 1918; 65:1180.

32   Hertoghe E. *Thyroid deficiency*. Lecture presented to the International Surgical Congress at the New York Polyclinic School and Hospital, New York, New York. International Clinic Week. April 1914. (Copies available through The Broda O. Barnes M.D. Research Foundation: www.brodabarnes.org).

33 Guyton A. *Textbook of Medical Physiology*. Philadelphia: WB Saunders Company; 2000.

34 Wallace D. Mitochondrial DNA in aging and disease. *Scientific American*. August 1997.

35 Brucker-Davis F, Weintraub B, Skarulis M, Grace M, Benichou J, Hauser P, et al. Genetic and clinical features of 42 kindreds with resistance to thyroid hormone, The National Institutes of Health prospective survey. *Annals of Internal Medicine*. 1995; 123(8):572-583.

36 Ramsay I. *Thyroid Disease and Muscle Dysfunction*. William Heinemann Medical Books LTD.; 1974.

37 Starr P. *Hypothyroidism: An Essay on Modern Medicine*. Springfield, IL: Charles C. Thomas; 1954.

38 Silenkow HR, Refetoff S. Common Tests of thyroid function in serum. *JAMA*. 1967; 202:135.

39 DeGroot LJ, Stanbury JB. *The Thyroid and Its Diseases*. 4th ed. New York: John Wiley and Sons, Inc.; 1975.

40 Rea WJ. *Chemical Sensitivities: Principles and Mechanisms, Volume 1*. Boca Raton, FL: Lewis Publishers; 1992.

41 Rea WJ. Clinical manifestations of pollutant overload. In *Chemical sensitivity, Volume III*. Boca Raton: CRC Press, Inc.; 1996.

42 Rea W. Proceedings of the 21st Annual Symposium on Man and His Environment, American Academy of Environmental Medicine Meeting. Plano, Texas: Audio-Visual Tapes: 2003. (www.aehf.com)

43 Eggertsen R, Petersen K, Lundberg PA, Nystron E, Lindstedt G. Screening for thyroid disease in a primary care unit with a thyroid stimulating hormone assay with a low detection limit. *BMJ*. 1988; 297:1586.

44 Jarlov A E, Nygarrd B, Hegedus L, Hartling SG, Hansen JM. Observer variations in the clinical and laboratory evaluation of patients with thyroid dysfunction and goiter. *Thyroid*. 1998; 8(5):393-398.

45 Zulewski H, Müller B, Exer P, Miserez AR, Staub J. Estimation of tissue hypothyroidism by a new clinical score: Evaluation of patients with various grades of hypothyroidism and controls. Division of Endocrinology, Department of Medicine, University Hospital of Basel, Basel, Switzerland. *Journal of Clinical Endocrinology and Metabolism*. 1997; 82(3):771-776.

46 Hertoghe J, Baiser W V, Eeckhaut W. Thyroid insufficiency. Is thyroxine the only valuable drug? *Journal of Nutritional & Environmental Medicine*. 2001; 11:159-166.

47   Peterson MC, Holbrook JH, Hales DV, Smith NL, Staker LV. Contributions of the history, physical examination, and laboratory investigation in making medical diagnosis. *West J Med.* 1992; 156: 163-65.

48   Lisser H, Escamilla RF. *Atlas of Clinical Endocrinology: Including Text of Diagnosis and Treatment.* St. Louis: C.V. Mosby Company; 1957.

49   Ross DS, Moses AC, Garber J, Ross DS, Lee SL, et al, Serum osteocalcin in patients taking l- thryoxine who have subclinical hyperthyroidism. *Journal of Clinical Endocrinology and Metabolism.* 1991; 72(2):507-509.

50   Paul TL, Kerrigan J, Kelly AM, Braverman LE, Baran DT. Long-term L-thyroxine therapy is associated with decreased hip bone density in premenopausal women. *JAMA.* 1988; 259(21):3137-3141.

51   Wenzel K. Bone minerals and levothyroxine. *Lancet.* 1992; 340: 435- 436.

52   Franklin JA, Betteridge J, Daykin J, Holder R, Oates GD, et al. Long term thyroxine treatment and bone mineral density. *Lancet.* 1992, 340:9-13.

53   Muller CG, Bayley TA, Harrison JE, Tsang R. Possible limited bone loss with suppressive thyroxine therapy is unlikely to have clinical relevance. *Thyroid.* 1995; 5(2):81-87.

54   DeGroot LJ, Larsen PR, Hennemann G. *The Thyroid and Its Diseases.* 6th Ed. New York: Churchill Livingstone Inc.; 1996. Page 559.

55   Barnes BO, Barnes CW. *Hope for hypoglycemia.* Revised Ed. America Book Company; 1999.

56   Sonkin L. Therapeutic trials with thyroid hormones in chemically normal thyroid patients with myofascial pain and complaints suggesting mild thyroid insufficiency. *Journal of Back and Musculoskeletal Rehabilitation.* 1997; 8(83):85.

57   Zondek H, Wolfsohn G, Myxoedema and psychosis. *Lancet.* 1944; 2:438-439.

58   Kraus H. *Diagnosis and Treatment of Muscle Pain.* Chicago: Quintessence Publishing Co., Inc; 1988.

59   Travell JG, Simons DG. *Myofascia Pain and Dysfunction, the Trigger Point Manual.* Baltimore: Williams & Wilkins; 1983.

60   Fahr G. Myxedema heart. *JAMA.* 1925; 84(5):345-349.

61   Escamilla RF. *Laboratory Aids in Endocrine Diagnosis.* Charles C. Thomas; 1954.

62   Barnes BO. The treatment of menstrual disorders in general practice. *Arizona Medicine.* 1949; 6:33.

63   Jefferies WM. *Safe Uses of Cortisol.* 2nd Ed. Springfield: Charles C. Thomas Publishers Ltd.; 1996.

64   Lorscheider F, Vimy M, Summers A. Mercury exposure from silver tooth fillings: Emerging evidence questions a traditional dental paradigm. *FASEBJ*. 1995; 9:504-508.

65   Swaim LT. Chronic arthritis. *JAMA*. 1929; 93:259.

66   Hill SR, Forsham PH, Thorn GW. The effect of adrenocorticotropin and cortisone on thyroid function, thyroid-adrenocortical interrelationships. *The Journal of Clinical Endocrinology*. 1950; 10:1375.

67   Rea W. *Chemical Sensitivity: Sources of Total Body Load, Volume 2*. Boca Raton: Lewis Publishers; 1992.

68   Gordon T, Kannel WB. Premature mortality from coronary heart disease: The Framingham Study. *JAMA*. 1971; 215:1617-1625.

68   Fishberg AM, Arteriosclerosis in thyroid deficiency. *JAMA*. 1924; 82:463-464.

69   Gaby A. *Preventing and Reversing Osteoporosis: Every Women's Essential Guide*. Prima Publishing, Rockland California; 1994.

70   Kirch W, Schafii C. Misdiagnosis at a university hospital in 4 medical eras. *Medicine*. 1996; 75(1):29-40.

71   Jackson I, Cobb W. Why does anyone still use desiccated thyroid USP? *American Journal of Medicine*. 1978; 64:284-288.

72   Melleby A, Kraus H. *The Y's Way to a Healthy Back*. Piscataway, New Jersey: New Century Publishers, Inc.; 1982.

73   Pelter R. Selenium's got the power. *American Druggist*. 1999; 216(11):48-49.

74   Shorr E. An evaluation of the clinical applications of the vaginal smear method. *Journal of the Mount Sinai Hospital*. May-June 1945; XII(1):667-688.

75   Sonkin LS, Cohen EJ. Treatment of the menopause. *Modern Treatment*. 1968; 5(3):545-563.

76   Brownstein D. *The miracle of natural hormones*. 2nd ed. Medical Alternatives Press, Inc.; 1999.

77   Vliet EL. *Screaming to be Heard: Hormonal Connections Women Suspect . . . and Doctors Ignore*. New York: M. Evans and Company; 1995.

78   Rea W. *Chemical Sensitivity: Tools for Diagnosis and Methods of Treatment, Volume 4*. Boca Raton: CRC Press; 1996.

79   Kelly G. Peripheral metabolism of thyroid hormones: A review. *Alternative Medicine Review*. 2000; 5(4):306-333.

80   Howdeshell K. A model of the development of the brain as a construct of the thyroid system. *Environmental Health Perspectives*. 2002; 110(supp 3):337-348.

81   Brucker-Davis, F. Effects of environmental synthetic chemicals on thyroid function. *Thyroid*. 1998; 8(9):827-856.

82 Colborn T, Dumanoski D, Myers JP. *Our Stolen Future: Are We Threatening Our Fertility, Intelligence, and Survival?-A Scientific Detective Story.* New York: Penguin; 1997.

83 Solomon G, Weiss P, Owen B, Citron A. Healthy milk, healthy baby: Chemical pollution and mother's milk. National Resources Defense Council. Available at: http://www.nrdc.org/breastmilk/default.asp. Accessed March 4, 2007.

84 Latini G, De Felice C, Presta G, Del Vecchio A, Paris I, Ruggeri F, et al. In utero exposure to di-(2-ethylhexyl)-phthalate and human pregnancy duration. *Environmental Health Perspectives.* 2003. Available at: http://ehp.niehs.nih.gov/docs/2003/6202/abstract.html. Accessed May 4, 2003.

85 Duty SM, Silva MJ, Barr DB, Brock JW, Ryan L, Chen Z, et al. Phthalate exposure and human semen parameters. *Epidemiology.* 2003; 14:269-277.

86 Stapleton R. *Lead is a Silent Hazard.* New York: Walker Publishing Company; 1994.

87 Huseman CA, Moriarty CM, Angle CR. Childhood lead toxicity and impaired release of thyroid stimulation hormone. *Environ Res.* 1987; 42:524-533.

88 Canfield RL, Henderson CR Jr, Cory-Slechta DA, Cox C, Jusko TA, Lanphear BP. Intellectual impairment in children with blood lead concentrations below 10 ug per deciliter. *New England Journal of Medicine.* 2003; 348(16):1517-1526.

89 Mercury Study Report to Congress. U.S. Environmental Protection Agency. Available at: http://www.epa.gov/mercury/report.htm. Accessed December 15, 1997.

90 Patrick L. Mercury toxicity and antioxidants: Part 1: Role of glutathione and alpha-lipoic acid in the treatment of mercury toxicity. *Alternative Medicine Review.* 2002; 7(6):456-471.

91 Baumgartner A, Campos-Barros A. Thyroid hormones and depressive disorders-clinical overview and perspectives. Part 2. Thyroid hormones and the central nervous system-basic research. *Nervenarzt.* 1993; 64:11-20.

92 Chen YJ, Hsu CC. Effects of prenatal exposure to PCBs on the neurological function of children: A neuropsychological and neurophysiological study. *Developmental Medicine and Child Neurology.* 1994; 36:312-320.

93 Wondisford FE. Editorial: Thyroid hormone action beyond the receptor. *Journal of Clinical Endocrinology and Metabolism.* 1996; 81(12):4194-4195.

94 Kraus H, Eisenmenger-Weber S. Fundamental considerations of posture exercises. *Physiother Rev.* 1947; 27:361-368.

95 Weiss RE, Hayashi Y, Nagaya T, Petty KJ, Murata Y, Seo H, et al. Dominant inheritance of resistance to thyroid hormone not linked to defects in the thyroid hormone receptor alpha or beta genes may be due to a defective cofactor. *Journal of Clinical Endocrinology and Metabolism.* 1996; 81(12):4196-4203.

96 Haley B. The relationship of the toxic effects of mercury to exacerbation of the medical condition classified as Alzheimer's diseases. *Nordic Journal of Biological Medicine.* 2003.

97 Wassertheil-Smoller S, Hendrix S, Limacher M, Heiss G, Kooperberg C, Baird A, et al. Effect of estrogen plus progestin on stroke in postmenopausal women. The Women's Health Initiative in a randomized trial. *JAMA.* 2003; 289(20):2673-2684.

98 Ford E, Giles W, Dietz W. Prevalence of the metabolic syndrome among U.S. adults: Findings from the third national health and nutrition examination survey. *JAMA.* 2002; 287(3):356-359.

99 Brownstein D. *Iodine: Why You Need It, Why You Can't Live Without It.* 3rd. ed. Medical Alternatives Press; 2008.

100 Stuart JJ, Pacholok SM. *Could It Be B12? An Epidemic of Misdiagnoses.* Sanger, CA: Quill Driver Books/Word Dancer Press; 2006.

101 Scanlan TS, Suchland KL, Hart ME, Huang Y, Crossley DA II, et al. 3-Iodothyronamine is an endogenous rapid-acting derivative of thyroid hormone. *Nature Medicine.* 2004; 10(6):638-642.

102 Environmental Working Group. July 14, 2005. *Body burden - the pollution in newborns: A benchmark investigation of industrial chemicals, pollutants and pesticides in umbilical cord blood.* Retrieved from http://www.ewg.org/reports/bodyburden2/execsumm.php

103 Quigley MET. Pain management in women: Empowering the female from pain of hormonal changes. Available at: http://www.youtube.com/watch?v=zVJ2yyJB5wg. Accessed February 28, 2007.

104 Women's Health Initiative (WHI) Study. Reported by: National Institutes of Health (NIH). Available at: http://www.nhlbi.nih.gov/whi/. Accessed March 3, 2007.

105 Writing Group for the Women's Health Initiative Investigators. Risks and benefits of estrogen plus progestin in healthy postmenopausal women: Principal results form the Women's Health Initiative randomized controlled trial. *JAMA.* July 17, 2002; 288(3):321-333.

106 Kulacz R, Levy TE, Jones JE. *The Root of Disease: Connecting Dentistry and Medicine.* 2nd ed. Philadelphia, PA: Xlibris Corporation; 2006.

107 Derry D M. *Breast Cancer and Iodine.* Victoria BC, Canada: Trafford Publishing; 2003.

108   Derry, D. Regeneration of human scar tissue with topical iodine: A preliminary report-part 1 (Three years). *Thryoid Science.* 2008;3(6):CR1-9. Retrieved from http:// www.thyroidscience.com/ cases/contents.htm. Accessed January 8, 2009.

109   Derry, D. Regeneration of human scar tissue with topical iodine: A preliminary report-part 2. *Thryoid Science.* 2008;3(7):CR1-9. Retrieved from http:// www.thyroidscience.com/cases/contents. htm. Accessed January 8, 2009.

Index